Leadership in Speech-Language Pathology

Leadership in Speech-Language Pathology

Linda S. Carozza, PhD, CCC-SLP

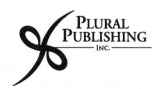

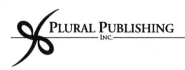

5521 Ruffin Road
San Diego, CA 92123

e-mail: information@pluralpublishing.com
Website: http://www.pluralpublishing.com

Library of Congress Cataloging-in-Publication Data

Names: Carozza, Linda S., author.
Title: Leadership in speech-language pathology / Linda S. Carozza.
Description: San Diego, CA : Plural Publishing, [2019] | Includes
   bibliographical references and index.
Identifiers: LCCN 2019001896| ISBN 9781944883614 (alk. paper) | ISBN
   1944883614 (alk. paper)
Subjects: | MESH: Speech-Language Pathology | Leadership
Classification: LCC RC425 | NLM WL 21 | DDC 616.85/5207—dc23
LC record available at https://lccn.loc.gov/2019001896

Contents

Introduction

The inspiration for this book came from many sources, such as life experience, opportunity, and happenstance. The lesson learned was that one can never be fully prepared for everything that will be necessary to lead a thriving group of professionals. Although this book endeavors to describe the major leadership qualities and resources to respond to those needs, the nature of interpersonal management of professionals in a fast-paced environment leaves many questions unanswered. The goal of the authors is to prepare as strong a landscape as possible so that hands-on learning, educational experience, and life skills work together to form a strategic whole.

When working with professionals, leaders encounter vast differences in experiences, values, and other variables of human interaction. The chapters in this book guide readers through self-discovery and a larger world view that together, will strengthen the preparedness of new and seasoned leaders. Overall, many of the insights emanate from a common stem; that is, the importance of adopting and integrating business and professional practices to work for the common good of an organization and its mission. Leadership is a heavy mantle to bear; a cornerstone of combined wisdom will provide a sense of the continuous journey that all leaders are on. Leaders hope to leave the environment where they worked and achieved success a better place for having been there. Reading, preparing, life experience, and if possible, the mentorship of a successful role model are all ingredients for what is essentially self-study of your strengths and weaknesses and how to respond to challenge.

In addition, working with a specialized group of leaders, like those in communications and related fields, presents unique circumstances to encounter and overcome. In a relatively young profession, role models are still developing and ever-changing, as the educational and medical landscape becomes increasingly complex. The talents and skills of new manager-leaders will be tested, and an understanding of the big picture, individual preparedness, and unknown quantities create a learning trajectory for new senior appointees. Whether learning by experience or modeling others' behavior, new leaders must develop a personal style based on knowledge of the industry, self-knowledge of ethics, and mastery of principles of fairness, consideration, design, and growth. Most environments do not allow for a long learning curve and new managers will be challenged early on unless they arrive with a strong skill set, and ego!

I am excited to go on a journey of discovery with emergent leaders in rehabilitation and allied fields. The material in the book was culled from many distinct perspectives over a period of time and reflects a journey of ongoing discovery that mindful leaders invariably undertake. From theory to practice to resource-finding, the chapters will guide professionals in areas that will likely reach beyond specific professional expertise. Emerging leaders should recognize and explore growth opportunities before being confronted with a wake-up call that an aspect of management in their unit is underperforming due to lack of preparedness for the distinct need for data and data management that could have forestalled unfortunate circumstances.

Above all, one aspires to become a competent and confident professional and to have the support of a well-earned reputation and achievement. In the words of many, happiness at work is a fulfillment that all of us seek. Knowing when something is a "want" as opposed to a "need" and avoidance of black-and-white all-or-nothing thinking are just two of the cognitive functions that leaders need to incorporate in their daily arsenal. Thomas Slominski, founder of Northern Speech services, recently published "Habits of Happy People." A well-known senior speech-language pathologist, Slominski discussed many insightful strategies needed to tackle high demand leadership and decision making, and the basic fact that people need to have insight to be concerned, but not overly worried, about work and goals. Lack of leadership and efficiency may be an issue of personality and background, as opposed to training and discipline in a specific field, and we address this issue in forthcoming chapters.

The American ideal of leadership espoused by the U.S. military bears mention in that there are multiple and potentially disparate perspectives on success, although many share very familiar themes. Peter Economy (2015) describes several strategies, listed below, that work for leadership in the military and that can also work in public and private industry.

1. Meeting the standard will always suffice if you want to be average or just get by. Exceeding the standard and living to a higher standard can lead to success and achieving your dreams.
2. Believe in something! Believe in yourself, believe in a creed, believe in your passion.
3. Heroes are everyday, ordinary people who have done something extraordinary. Honor them, praise them, and hope that like them, you will stand for what you believe in during times of need.
4. Be disciplined. Know what right looks like.
5. Never walk by a mistake, or you just set a new lower standard!
6. Invincibility is a myth. Recognize and optimize your strengths and deal with your weaknesses to minimize them.
7. Don't stop trying or fighting for what you believe in the first time someone tells you "no."
8. Don't compromise your principles.
9. People are always watching you. What you do sets the tone for others.
10. Have the guts—courage—to do the right thing for the right reason.
11. The best way to have healthy debates and find the ultimate solutions to very complex problems is to have the best and brightest group of people to offer diverse perspectives on the issues. Be inclusive, not exclusive; embrace diversity of thought in management and in key leadership teams.
12. Build high-performing teams or organizations. Build teams that routinely do routine things in an outstanding manner.
13. Provide a strategic vision. Visualize where you want your team to be in the future and design a roadmap to get there. It is key that *all* individuals in your organization understands how important they are to accomplishing the vision.

14. Enjoy your job and make a difference. Some of the most difficult decisions we make in our lives center around deciding how long to stay, when to change, or when to leave. Don't leave these decisions to someone else or to chance—make them *your* decisions.

Not many people will be in a high-command position in the military, but the principles cited have great similarity to other leadership literature. In "Leadership Strategies to Help You Handle Change" (http://www.superperformance.com), Kathleen O'Connor speaks about the gathering information, building a subordinate staff ready to move up, knowing your job, and what you need to know to do your job. On this point, expectations or job descriptions for leaders and their staff are critical. In times of change, these may be a moving target, and it is vital that manager-leaders have the cooperation and insight from the highest level of administration in the organization so everyone is on the same page. Change is hard for individuals, but buy-in and team engagement and empowerment, even in difficult times, can be achieved if sufficient groundwork is laid. That can take the shape of a team retreat or reading a related article, and can include many other points of team satisfaction. O'Connor cautions that leaders should change before they have to, and should be aware that environments evolve quickly, so that they can anticipate and plan for change. To this end, using consultants, such as managerial coaches, can help leaders understand and master change outside of the fixed work environment, as well as empower new professionals.

In the search for work and understanding in academic and health leadership, there are a plethora of writings, meetings, and opportunities to learn. Finding resources that will enhance an organization that all leaders aspire to is a complex task. Through readings and participating in and leading professional seminars, I have found that the *Harvard Business Review* speaks to some of the important matters at the heart of leadership. Their online "Tips of the Day" are useful for the daily discipline that being a manager entails, emphasizing that leadership deals with the details of human dynamics, in addition to work products.

To this end, the commonality and strength of the principles put forth by professionals, such as those at Wharton and other leading institutions, have consistent tenets. Leitch, Lancefield, and Dawson (2016) stress that challenging without provocation, attention to the big picture as well as the details, willingness to change course of action, and leading with engagement and respect are essential qualities of lasting leadership. The goal of transparency and the possibility that there are multiple paths to a goal are additional ideals in the workplace that will grow and flourish (https://www.strategy-business.com/article/10-Principles-of-Strategic-Leadership).

The question remains then, with so much information, and much of it strikingly similar in ideals and tone, why is leadership so often a role with quick turnover, causing organizations to lose momentum and the footing to move forward in strategic plans and long-term goals? Questions like this inspired the work in this book. All change on a personal, professional, or organizational level is a process. If an organization is willing to invest in a professional as a leader, there is a growth curve, along with some detours, that a dedicated professional must conquer.

Undoubtedly, readers of this book are among those who turn the lens inward, as well as outward to prevailing wisdom and literature, to be the best professionals they can be. It will be a reward if the new ideas that evolve from this book can be reflected in forthcoming work and collaborations among emergent leaders in the field.

References

Economy, P. (2015, April 13). *15 Leadership strategies from America's first female 4-star general.* Retrieved from https://www.inc.com/peter-economy/15-leadership-strategies-from-america-s-first-female-4-star-general.html

Leitch, J., Lancefield, D., & Dawson, M. (2016, May 18). *10 Principles of strategic leadership.* Retrieved from https://www.strategy-business.com/article/10-Principles-of-Strategic-Leadership?gko=25cec

Acknowledgments

This book is based on the incredible inspired teamwork and vision of my immediate collaborators, Tanya Radison and Noel Shafi. The work of these inspirational young professionals allowed me to begin this journey of self-discovery to share with others who are walking or will walk the same path. Likewise, my contributing authors, Wendy Papir-Bernstein, Regina Lemmon-Bush, and Katie LaForce, are among the most amazing and generous colleagues I could have had the good fortune to meet on this journey. Professor Bernstein's in-depth and masterful review of diverse components of leadership will help shape the viewpoints of many future colleagues. Likewise, meeting Dr. Lemmon-Bush and her team was a turning point for me, and I was inspired by her from the moment we encountered our like-mindedness at an ASHA convention not too long ago and developed a friendship and kinship. I can only hope that her vision for leadership and change will enlighten the path of many professionals to come.

I have also had the extreme gift of support and advocacy from the professionals at Plural Publishing. With two books beforehand, I knew I would be in good hands and I am humbled by their confidence in me to develop and write on leadership, as my books have followed my life's journey, so to speak.

Many other colleagues, students, and friends have accompanied me throughout my career as I aspire to do for them. I have learned so much and every day, wake up with a thirst for how I can do something better. My career in speech-language pathology has been one of my greatest gifts, helping me, as I hope I have helped others. The work of a book has many voices and influences and I am deeply grateful to all who have spoken to me and shared insight on their own experiences and careers. It is my hope that this book engenders even more conversations on why and how to lead when the time is right in your career.

Contributors

Linda S. Carozza, PhD, CCC-SLP
Founding Director, MS Program in Communication Sciences and Disorders
Pace University
Clinical Assistant Professor
Department of Rehabilitation Medicine
New York University Langone Medical Center
New York, New York
Chapters 1, 2, 3, 4, 5, 6, and 7

Katie LaForce, BA, CCC-SLP
Research Specialist I
University of South Carolina, MSP 2020
Undergraduate Matriculation
Columbia College
Columbia, South Carolina
Chapter 7

Regina Lemmon-Bush, PhD, CCC-SLP
Program Chair and Associate Professor
Speech-Language Pathology
Columbia College
Past President
South Carolina Speech Language Hearing Association (SCSHA)
Columbia, South Carolina
Chapter 10

Wendy Papir-Bernstein, CCC-SLP
ASHA Fellow
Associate Professor, Adjunct
Lehman College, CUNY
Retired Speech Supervisor NYCDOE D75
President-Elect
New York State Speech-Language-Hearing Association (NYSSLHA)
New York, New York
Chapters 8 and 9

Reviewers

Celia R. Hooper, PhD
Dean Emeritus
School of Health and Human Sciences
Professor, Communication Sciences and Disorders
University of North Carolina Greensboro
Greensboro, North Carolina

Stephanie O'Silas, MS, CCC-SLP
Champion Rehabilitation and Support Services PLLC
Director of Therapy & Engagement
Dallas, Texas

Judith O. Roman, MA, CCC-SLP, BRS-CL
Clinical Faculty
Northwestern University
Evanston, Illinois

Donna Fisher Smiley, PhD, CCC-A
Audiology Supervisor
Arkansas Children's Hospital
Little Rock, Arkansas

Jane R. Wegner, PhD, CCC-SLP
Director, Schiefelbusch Speech-Language-Hearing Clinic
University of Kansas
Lawrence, Kansas

I dedicate this book to my loved ones. Gabriel Alexander, I hope you grow and thrive to be master of your fate and that all you endeavor and wish for will come true.

1

Why Study Leadership?

Linda S. Carozza

The art of communication is the language of leadership.
—James Humes

Learning Objectives

- Readers will gain awareness on the issue of leadership in the professional development of speech-language pathology practitioners.
- Readers will be introduced to the following chapters as they relate to identification of skills and methodologies to attain these leadership abilities.

Call for Action

Speech-language pathology is one of the fastest growing health professions, with a projected increase in growth of 18% between 2016 to 2026 (Bureau of Labor Statistics, 2017). The growth of the profession stems from a number of factors, including a rapid increase in aging populations, medical advances that improve the survival rate of preterm infants, as well as trauma and stroke patients, growth in elementary and secondary school enrollments, and increasing demand in health care and private practice settings (American Speech-Language-Hearing Association [ASHA], 2017). This growth of the field, while great for yielding more jobs and more opportunities for individuals and families to receive much needed services and support, also means an increase in the roles and responsibilities of speech-language pathologists (SLPs), including managerial or leadership roles within their respective organizations.

Whereas moving up the career ladder is typically seen as the ultimate end goal in most professions, one of the main challenges for SLPs in advancing is a lack of sufficient training and preparation (Kummer, 2017). Because speech pathology is at its core a clinically-based health profession, the majority of training and experience revolves around gaining an understanding of the typically developing processes of communication (including speech, language, and hearing) and training in the prevention, assessment, diagnosis, and treatment of communication disorders (ASHA, 2017). Kummer (2017) posits that leadership is an inherent quality and characteristic of our profession and states that "in clinical situations, we lead; we guide our patients and their family members; in supervisory situations, we lead and guide our employees and students; in professional situations, with colleagues and coworkers, we lead and guide on a daily basis" (p. 1).

Nevertheless, such constructs still require a more complex set of skills and abilities when compared to leadership on a larger scale. Many SLPs rise to management and leadership positions within their organizations, but without having had opportunities for formal continuing education in management and leadership skills which are often acquired through on-the-job training, mentoring, and continuing professional education (ASHA, 2003). Thus, many clinicians may find themselves ill-equipped and unprepared to take on larger roles which are less reliant on the clinical skills in which they were trained.

Thus, this book serves as a much needed guide for addressing workplace challenges that confront managerial, supervisory, and leadership professionals in the field of communication sciences and disorders (CSD). The premise and inspiration for this book is based on words of wisdom for leaders, given to me long ago by one of the wisest people I ever knew, my former mentor.

Those words of wisdom, based on his long-standing career as a beloved leader in the military, consisted of two questions for self-reflection that he relied on whenever we discussed life and workplace issues: "Did you do the best you could do?" and "Did you tell the truth?" He told me that if people can answer "yes" to both of these questions, they would always be able to face any issue they encountered.

Need for More Effective Leadership

From my years of experience, it appears that the field tends to rely on internal sources to fill managerial positions. In many cases, the same applies for supervisory and directorship titles. Although it certainly makes sense to work with professionals whose experience and integrity you are familiar with and can trust, this at times presents the newly promoted with a quandary in terms of resources. Although ASHA provides a number of professional resources for managing a new business practice, there is little scholarship directed toward the specifics of developing or establishing a CSD program within a structure that has pre-existing and collateral units. Such specifics include needs analysis, stepwise planning for program development and expansion, and a plan for establishing a long-term presence. These are very significant undertakings requiring thought, practice, experience, and often, time-sensitive actions that must occur simultaneously with the delivery of effective services to the public. In viewing this dearth of leadership and management skills training for clinical SLPs through the additional lens of curriculum/program development, it is important to remember that leadership in higher education presents a unique set of challenges as compared to leadership in other settings (Buller, 2013).

When SLPs are in the midst of developing new programs or carrying forward and enhancing the visions of others, they may find themselves thinking about evidence-based approaches and looking to the literature. In doing so myself, I noticed a scarcity of data on how to effectively develop and nurture a program via planned leadership practice. I consider leadership a hot topic in the establishment of best practices in speech-language pathology, which is an emerging area of research interest within the field.

In fact, even the naming of a unit or department takes a depth of knowledge that may be obscure to younger or untrained leaders. I consider effective leadership to be something that we owe our fellow practitioners, scientists, administrators, and faculty members.

Defining Leadership

In preparing for this book, I needed to develop a sense of how *leadership* is defined in the general marketplace. As it turns out, there exist a plethora of constructs and definitions for the term, making it somewhat difficult to clearly characterize, particularly as it relates to various disciplines and contexts. According to Ledlow and Stephens (2018), the following definition can be used specifically for health leaders:

> The dynamic and active creation and maintenance of an organizational culture and strategic systems that focus the collective energy of both leading people and managing resources toward meeting the needs of the external environment utilizing the most efficient, effective, and efficacious methods possible by moral means. (p. 14)

In short, the distinction between leadership in other fields, as opposed to health care, comes from the inclusion of patient needs (external environment) and the overarching ethical standards of the Hippocratic Oath. Furthermore, it is important to distinguish between the terms leadership and management, as the two are at times used interchangeably, leading to a blurred distinction. Management refers to a role which is "more reactive and remains closely coupled with organizational policies, standards, guidelines, and established processes," whereas a health leader is more "proactive, involved in developing the organizational culture and strategic systems necessary to maximize the efficiency, effectiveness, and efficacy of the organization within the external environment" (Ledlow & Stephens, 2018, p. 14).

Kummer (2017) further specifies that the term *leadership* is not job specific, but rather, situation specific.

In the field of speech-language pathology, examples of situations in which clinicians may demonstrate leadership roles include the following: clinical supervisor, mentor to new colleagues, committee chair, advocate for legislative change, and team leader in patients' plan of care (Kummer, 2017). Parallels exist between SLPs acting in a clinical capacity and leaders of corporations and organizations—namely, that the overall goals and processes are very similar in both contexts. As outlined by Kummer (2017), the primary and most important task for the leader of an organization is the development of a vision. Vision is further defined as the creation of an idea of where the leader will take the organization, and what the organization will look like in the future. The second most important task is the subsequent development of strategic goals to accomplish said vision (Kummer, 2017).

This directly parallels the process of working with clients, which necessitates developing both long-term goals focused on improving overall speech, language, and communication skills, as well as short-term goal plans aimed at helping clients attain said goals over a specified time span. Thus, clinicians may already possess part of the framework needed to develop into strong and effective leaders. Leadership qualities are demonstrated in long- versus short-term planning on considerably different scales, and each requires explicit training and education.

In addition to explicitly defining leadership and the specific contexts in which it can be demonstrated, we must also consider the actual qualities and characteristics that make someone an effective leader. We intend to contribute our point of view on what makes for a poor leader, which is a yardstick for reflecting on the polar opposite qualities hopefully found in good leaders. Though poor leadership may be less apparent during a period of growth in an organization, a lack of leadership is very marked when an organization goes through lean times for any variety of reasons. Zenger and Folkman (2009) looked back at 360-degree feedback data for more than 11,000 executives and identified 10 leadership shortcomings, among them "not walking the talk," failing to learn from mistakes, and lacking a clear vision and direction. Other leadership flaws include difficulties with challenge, lack of collaboration, resistance to input, failure to develop colleagues' potential, and lack of insightful communicative behaviors. The authors propose that owing to these leadership flaws, employees are left with a sense of abandonment of group purpose and collective mission.

Although some individuals possess natural tendencies toward leadership qualities and perhaps are described by others as natural born leaders, effective leadership nevertheless requires a great deal of training and practice. The prospect of assuming a leadership position undoubtedly comes with a great burden of responsibility and can seem very daunting for someone whose primary qualification may be knowledge and experience in their specific field or discipline, yet has limited or no hands-on leadership training (Nawaz, 2017). With particular application to the field of CSD, ASHA provides a list of specific knowledge, skills, and competencies needed by organizational managers and leaders to fulfill their roles as they pertain to business practices underlying service delivery in health care (ASHA, 2003).

Challenges of Leadership

Astin and Astin (2006), in *Leadership Reconsidered: Engaging Higher Education in Social Change,* speak to many of the underlying factors that confront the development of future leaders. First, young academics may not be familiar with the notion that institutions of higher education are the driving forces of social change and development in Western society. Second, that higher education-led societal change is most organic when the roles of individual constituents (students, educators, administrators) are considered collectively/as part of an integrated whole. Unfortunately, this is not yet a goal on many agendas due to the unfortunate and more pressing societal concerns of safety, survival, and equality. Third, faculty and program directors, department chairs, and high-level administrators, need to recognize the role of educational, medical, and health institutions in affecting social change to meet the needs of the future. Health professions face additional and unique leadership challenges including the enormous size of the industry, unaligned motivations, scarcity of resources, and lack of a unifying and widely accepted vision (Ledlow & Stephens, 2018). Organizational leaders in the health care fields have a unique opportunity to influence not only health-related, but other institutions as well.

Need for Effective Leadership Training

How did leadership emerge as an area of need and growth in our profession? Despite the fact that the CSD field has long been a profession disproportionately populated by women (Maier, 2013) with master's-level preparedness, there is little opportunity for hands-on learning in an organization, and even less student-level preparation (even in the doctoral programs) for eventual lead roles in service delivery or academic departments. Furthermore, although there is increasing longevity in the field and opportunity for expansion and advancement, there is still a lack of lack of options to obtain credentials for managerial and directorial positions. As an example, in the current medical economy where results and accountability must be addressed in the planning stages, it is essential for new directors to have knowledge of the national landscape, student trends, and allied professional fields. Leaders also need to know how to position a department for visibility and growth out of the gate. In order to take a seat at the table with a board of directors or other senior executives, new managers must demonstrate both personal and professional leadership capacity.

The concept of leadership and the educational goals of leadership development have been given little attention by most of institutions of higher learning. It seems to be the case that in classrooms, faculty continue to emphasize the acquisition of knowledge in traditional disciplinary fields and the development of writing, quantitative, and critical thinking skills, giving relatively little attention to developing personal qualities that are most crucial to effective leadership: self-understanding, listening skills, empathy, honesty, integrity, and the ability to work collaboratively. According to Astin and Astin (2006), leadership qualities in modern American society are in large part shaped and influenced by higher education, the role of which is multi-faceted. Higher education not only educates each new generation of leaders but also sets curriculum standards, trains future personnel, and influences leadership practices through research and scholarship, which seek to clarify the meaning, method, and training of leadership and to identify the most effective approaches to leadership and leadership education.

Some organizations in our profession, such as the Council of Academic Programs in Communication Sciences and Disorders (CAPCSD), provide leadership training because they recognize the need for leadership development, renewal, and succession; however, these opportunities may be limited to annual training and may be more generalized than is ideal. Therefore, the ability to have access to one's own resources at will significantly supports directors in charge of the ongoing needs of a department. I believe that SLPs who are devoted to scholarship and evidence-based practice want to perform at their highest level and take their rightful leadership roles. The fact that departments depend on financial viability makes effective and knowledgeable leadership essential in order for programs to survive. Furthermore, as stated in *Nonprofit Sustainability: Making Strategic Decisions for Financial Viability,*

> financial sustainability and programmatic sustainability cannot be separated. It's not enough to have a high-impact program if there's no effective strategy for sustaining the organization financially. And neither is it enough to be financially stable; we build our organizations for impact, not for financial stability. Yet surprisingly, in the nonprofit sector, financial information and information about mission impact are seldom discussed in an integrated way. (Bell, Masaoke, & Zimmerman, 2010, p. 3)

Challenges in Accepting Leadership

The discussions herein span settings including schools, universities, hospitals, private practices, rehabilitation agencies, and many other organizations. In each setting, a group of professionals must make decisions about what is important in each community of service and how to conduct business. Establishing rules of practice for planned and unplanned situations comprise the art and science of effective leadership. As new leaders, senior managers or directors may find themselves in need of leadership onboarding, coaching, and ongoing training. However, within CSD, in addition to a lack of managerial and senior-level administration training from within the profession, there is little use of established training practices from other professions.

This book is written for those who may have learned on the job or just learned on the job and seek more up-front preparation on the various aspects that are encompassed by leadership endeavors. This includes big picture foundational concepts, such as developing mission, vision, and strategic planning for oneself as an individual, one's department and overall organization, as well as for smaller-scale day-to-day objectives, such as self-growth, business practices, time and stress management, and learning to build bridges, resolve conflict, and when and how to say "no."

Longevity in CSD

According to Astin and Astin (2006), a major problem with contemporary civic life in America is that too few citizens are actively engaged in effecting positive social change. Viewed in this context, an important leadership development challenge for higher education is to empower students to develop the special talents and attitudes that will enable them to become effective social change agents. This is both an individual and an institutional challenge. Students will find it difficult to lead until they have experienced effective leadership as part of their education. They are not likely to commit to making changes in society unless their training institutions display a similar commitment. If the next generation of citizen leaders is to be engaged and committed to leading for the common good, then the institutions that nurture them must be engaged in working for society and the community, modeling effective leadership and problem-solving skills, and demonstrating how to accomplish social change. This requires institutions of higher education to set their own house in order, if they expect to produce students who will improve society.

Culture of Civility

The role of civility in academe has been a hot button topic for many years. As described by Nigel Thrift in the *Chronicle of Higher Education* (2014), we have progressed from a past where academic leadership was considered similar to a feudal society in which only favored, younger protégés received opportunity and advancement. In defining civility as a respect and consideration for all (i.e., inclusivity), it becomes clear how important it is in a discussion about academic leadership and promotion. A more civil academic culture, one that solicits and respects viewpoints from all members regardless of role, leads to overall progression, growth, and realization of vision. Growth in this arena has occurred in recent years. Increased public awareness and diversity, and more opportunities in the academic pipeline have contributed to the establishment of streamlined and consistent decisions about qualifications for promotion to leadership positions.

When educational issues enter the political sphere (as they often do) it means that these struggles are far from over, although owing to it there may be more of a public venue or access to academic decisions in some instances.

An important concept related to civility is its breakdown in academic and training environments, despite concentrated efforts to bring civility training into the workplace. The notion of individuals struggling alone is prominent in the high stakes environment of today's economy. As a profession, the field of CSD has a great deal of inherent competition—from grades, to spots in graduate school programs, to desired job placements, spanning all the way to overall competition in the workplace. In fact, civility, if it is not measured and delivered carefully, can instead be seen as a sign of meekness. Thrift (2014) points out that many senior faculty may treat new administrators with a lack of dignity and respect, while at the same time depending on them to arrange availability, arrange public information, and arrange other critical factors that recruit and retain students. This issue becomes more challenging when the administrators share the same academic discipline as the faculty they work with or lead.

Trending

Chapter 2 discusses the qualities of effective leadership from many broad perspectives and the chapters that follow develop discussion points raised in this introduction.

Reflection

Think about your training as an SLP. Did any of your coursework emphasize leadership training of any sort?

References

American Speech-Language-Hearing Association. (2003). *Knowledge and skills in business practices for speech-language pathologists who are managers and leaders in health-care organizations.* Retrieved from http://www.asha.org/policy/KS2004-00073.htm

American Speech-Language-Hearing Association. (2017). *Speech-language pathologists.* Retrieved from http://www.asha.org/Students/Speech-Language-Pathologists/

Astin, A., & Astin, S. (2006). *Leadership reconsidered: Engaging higher education in social change.* Retrieved from http://www.naspa.org/images/uploads/kcs/SLPKC_Learning_Reconsidered.pdf

Bureau of Labor Statistics, Occupational Outlook Handbook, 2017. Retrieved from https://www.bls.gov/ooh/healthcare/speech-language-pathologists.htm

Bell, J., Masaoke, J., & Zimmerman, S. (2010). *Nonprofit sustainability: Making strategic decisions for financial viability.* New York, NY: Wiley.

Buller, J. (2014). *Change leadership in higher education: A practical guide to academic transformation.* San Francisco, CA: Jossey-Bass.

Kummer, A. (2017, January 17). Leadership and the art of influencing others [Transcript of webinar]. *SpeechPathology.com*. Retrieved from https://www.speechpathology.com/articles/leadership-and-art-influencing-others-18980

Ledlow, G., & Stephens, J. (2018). *Leadership for health professionals: Theory, skills, and applications* (3rd ed.). Burlington, MA: Jones & Bartlett Learning.

Maier, K. (2013, August 13) Why the scarcity of male SLPs—and what can be done [Blog post]. Retrieved from http://blog.asha.org/2013/08/13/why-the-scarcity-of-male-slps-and-what-can-be-done/

Nawaz, S. (2017, May 15) The biggest mistakes new executives make. *Harvard Business Review*. Retrieved from https://hbr.org/2017/05/the-biggest-mistakes-new-executives-make

Thrift, N. (2014, April 15). Civility in academe, and the lack of it [Blog post]. Retrieved from http://www.chronicle.com/blogs/worldwise/civility-in-academe-and-the-lack-of-it/33395

Zenger, J., & Folkman, J. (2009, June). Ten fatal flaws that derail leaders. *Harvard Business Review*. Retrieved from https://hbr.org/2009/06/ten-fatal-flaws-that-derail-leaders

Additional Resources

Davis, J. (1992) In praise of civility. *American Journal of Audiology*, *1*(2), 7. https://doi.org/10.1044/1059-0889.0102.07

Economy, P. (2013, August 27). 7 traits of highly effective leaders. *Inc*. Retrieved from: https://www.inc.com/peter-economy/7-traits-highly-effective-leaders.html

2

Qualities of Effective Leaders

Linda S. Carozza

Before you are a leader, success is all about growing yourself. When you become a leader, success is all about growing others.

—Jack Welch

Learning Objective

- To describe the literature pertaining to the professional qualities ascribed to leadership potential, which relate to either the skill development that takes place during academic and clinical training; or to characteristics of personality and more innate nonacquired leadership skills.

Think Question

What are some character traits or qualities that make someone a great leader?

Introduction

This chapter is an effort to gather the insights of senior leaders in the allied health and education professions to learn about leadership from their vantage point and experience. Readers will get a glimpse into some of the important lessons that cannot be gained from books or in a classroom, but rather, are learned from experience, time, and energy spent managing and developing teams and programs. These insights and experiences are based on evidence in the literature and interviews with senior health care leaders about rewards and challenges experienced during their careers.

Core Competencies for Leadership Potential

Pilling and Slattery (2004) examined the perceived competencies that underlie career transitions to management that stretch beyond one's basic educational training. They hypothesized that certain SLP competencies are transferable to management and even to senior health management roles.

For the purposes of their study, conducted in Australia, competence was operationally defined. They note that although standard definitions abound, ultimately, competence is more than a set of behavioral skills. The idea that competence evolves in different circumstances and as needs change is one that has flexibility to encompass both threshold competence and the mature competence that emerges with organizational culture and change. This growth can be enhanced and facilitated through conscious strategies such as reflective practice, an approach that is well known in speech-pathology (Carozza, 2010).

Leadership qualities entail not only skills, but also personality traits and characteristics, which are more elusive to define and train. Core competencies identified in the Pilling and Slattery study were the ability to work with people, financial management, and interpersonal negotiation skills. Also, there are differing competencies required depending on whether a manager is in a middle- or senior-level position. Senior health care executives, for example, leaders responsible for a comprehensive rehabilitation department, require a deep understanding of how organizations develop and thrive in today's marketplace and of government regulations, and also require in-depth skills in demonstrating and developing outcomes and outcomes models.

Pilling and Slattery (2004) note that middle managers are more concerned with maintaining and supervising workflow, whereas senior managers design and develop new programs and offerings and establish the related policies. The high-level managers are tasked with objectives that may be more amorphous, calling for work with more vision and creativity for the future, whereas middle managers are called upon to direct more concrete day-to-day operations.

Overall, the managers queried reported six skills as the most vital for successfully transitioning to administration: (1) effective communication skills, (2) problem-solving ability, (3) a commitment to evidence-based practice and accountability, (4) teamwork skills, (5) focus, and (6) background in health care.

According to the authors, most management training takes place outside of a formal classroom and involves both practical and hands-on experiential training. This finding is supported easily with real-world examples of promotions to management positions without the requisite official training or degree (such as an MBA). There is reason to believe that the skills of a good clinician involve management and delivery of a product, but logically speaking managing a department presents different challenges than managing clinical disorders per se. Interestingly, SLPs move up the ranks almost exclusively through informal networks and on the job training. When a career transitions, individuals must identify required transformational needs that. This mental shift necessitates that individuals move out of their comfort zone.

After identifying the six aforementioned skills, Pilling and Slattery questioned whether these skills were intrinsic in speech-language pathology professionals. However, their study was unable to delineate which skills were inherent for clinicians and which were acquired after their initial professional training.

The study concluded that overall, skills in human resource management, administration and leadership, and finance and strategy were considered underdeveloped in newly promoted clinicians. The fact that clinicians are trained to be empathic was seen as a downside to the administrative mindset by many respondents. Another factor that was brought to light is that frequently, advancement may be limited for SLPs because the small number on staff makes them disadvantaged when compared to other professionals who account for a larger proportion of the staff. A good example is that rehab departments are more typically managed by physical therapists than SLPs, because physical therapists have greater visibility than SLPs in rehab departments, leading to more promotions for physical therapists. Another important consideration is that many senior clinicians, regardless of field, may feel pressure to advance in their career as opposed to being seen as stagnant or stale, and so clinicians may take on a role primarily out of seniority factors, and not because of an inherent skill set.

Pilling and Slattery's (2004) interviewees rated the role of formal education as critical in leadership skills. Ideologies pertaining to less formal training, such as mentorship and simply learning on the job, are no longer as sufficient as they may have been in the past. The overall consensus was that moving from a senior speech pathologist position to program director, administrator, and related titles constitutes a career change. The authors cited several studies in which fiscal management training is specifically needed in order to succeed (Fine, 2002; Hartman & Crow, 2002). Managers who identify primarily with their clinical field later experience feeling unempowered, undue job pressure, and paralysis in their new role. It is primarily for these reasons that clinician-managers must seek allied training, such as continuing education in health care, administrative seminars, and certificate programs prior to and early in their administrative careers.

Managers in the Pilling and Slattery (2004) study were called by different titles depending on their organization. Using different titles can obscure a comparison of duties, levels of responsibility, and the specificity of previous training; whether that training be on the job, formal academic education or specialized curriculum designed for managers. Titles used in that study included general manager, university lecturer, program director, senior quality manager, allied health director, management consultant, executive office, operations director, human resources director, and university course coordinator. In addition, years since graduation from a clinical training program and years in a management position varied greatly across their respondents, which may confound the reliability of survey results.

These types of methodological issues are common in leadership studies because some managers are promoted from within and others are graduates of formal training programs. However, Pilling and Slattery (2004) method of contemporaneous interviewing and fact-finding is an important initial attempt to grasp a problem with many diverse factors.

Gardner (1999) developed a five-skill hierarchy of aptitudes vital for leadership positions. They are: intrapersonal awareness, interpersonal awareness, supporting others, managing others, and organization and environmental awareness. Gardner contends that these skills emerge over time as managers mature and take on roles with increasing responsibility. However, his position is controversial, as others believe that managers are born, not made, and that the five aforementioned skills are more intrinsic or innately personality based. According to Goleman (2004), one of the most important qualities shared by great leaders is emotional intelligence, including self-awareness, self-regulation, motivation, empathy, and social skills. Each of these qualities have been linked directly to strong performance based on measurable results (Goleman, 2004; Rao, 2006).

To develop an aptitude in organization/environmental awareness requires a 360-degree view of past, present, and future perspectives and inquiries. This encompasses more obvious or easily trackable items such as the pre-existing setup of an organization and the way it was developed and managed; the current working model and issues within the model; how to best respond to problems; and ways in which to prevent problems from reoccurring. However, this 360-degree view should also encompass more mutable/less trackable items that occur in a work environment, such as organizational culture and pre-existing power structures and alliances. All of these factors can be seen as a virtual minefield that can temper the ambitions of novices with little prior experience, even before their leadership skills ever have a chance to fully form and mature.

Leadership Self-Assessment

The essential message from the participating leaders in the studies cited above, chosen for their experiences and diversity, is summarized below. A combination of personality, judgment, and directed education can produce a leader, and some individuals are naturally more inclined toward leadership than others. Many pitfalls can be avoided by learning specific skills before taking on senior responsibilities.

Many experts will say that leadership is all in how you present information. Thusly, as communication specialists, SLPs should intuitively be able to present information to enhance their leadership. This is, in a sense, overly simplistic in that it does not take into account the many preexisting histories that impact a group of people in an organization. If there is sufficient interest and financial backing in an organization to train new leaders, one of the first trainings that a new manager receives(either in a class or one-on-one) is usually a workshop on corporate communication. Although communication specialists can often instruct on concepts of leadership, many may not necessarily be good leaders themselves. It takes many skills and an array of professional communication prowess to be the kind of leader that inspires others to share a vision.

Self-assessment is one of the tools used by the Massachusetts Institute of Technology's Leader to Leader Program. This tool can be used by individuals in leadership positions to gauge their own strength and weakness and to improve self-awareness of specific skills that may need further development. Effective leadership requires an awareness of the interplay between interpersonal and intrapersonal factors as it relates to managing and making important decisions. Thus, it is crucial that good leaders are willing to be open, honest, and reflective when it comes to evaluating their own leadership style. Not only will this improve outcomes for the organization but it also sets a good model for employees and staff members by promoting an environment of personal growth and accountability.

Leadership Interviews

This following section includes interviews with senior academic leaders who shared their experiences to stimulate reflection on the principles of leadership. The interview questions were meant as a guide, but interviewees had free rein to discuss whatever they felt was important to say.

Interview #1

1. What do you perceive to be the most important traits or qualities of a good leader? Please explain their significance.

I am very familiar with the many different characteristics that make a good leader. I have experienced firsthand these leadership characteristics. Based on my experiences, the characteristics of leadership that I value the most are (1) communication, (2) commitment, and (3) decision-making and problem-solving.

First, I believe that good communication is an essential characteristic for any person in a leadership role. This is undisputed on many levels. The best leaders are those who excel when they are able to communicate with others or their team to move an agenda forward. They must be articulate and good listeners with the ability to communicate effectively with every level of a team or group. They should be able to motivate others and share their plan of action, their vision, and their ideas.

Second, I believe that commitment is the benchmark of leadership that complements communication—the ability to engage others to take ownership in the goals and mission of the team or group. You have to lead by example and be committed to achieve the goals set out. It is important for the team or group to see committed leaders roll up their sleeves and work just as hard as everyone on the team or group. When this is done, a good leader with a positive attitude will have inspired the team or group to be engaged in the mission at hand, which in turn will result in their loyalty and a win-win perspective for the team and the goals that they have set out to accomplish.

Last, but not least (as this list of characteristics can be lengthy), I believe that decision-making and problem-solving are the leadership qualities that have always resonated with the concept of true leadership. Decision-making and problem-solving go hand-in-hand; an effective leader must know how to make good decisions that may impact the group or organization or be able to resolve a problem with strategic thinking, analysis, and a decisive plan of action. Leaders with these qualities possess good foresight and sound judgment, especially under difficult and stressful, pressure-filled situations.

I believe these traits are essential to the makeup of a good leader. They are of vital importance because they provide an individual with the opportunity to become an agent of change; to influence others, to identify situations and problems, and provide solutions with the ultimate goal of achieving consensus. These leadership qualities are developed in an individual with every leadership opportunity they are confronted with. In order to be a leader, however, you have to make a conscious decision to be one and be prepared to lead; to lead others by example and to educate those around you; to seek buy-in on an objective or goal; to collaborate and to provide different perspectives on an issue or on how we do things that may influence or impact others.

2. What are some of the rewards and challenges of being a leader?

"You win by the sword and die by the sword." A successful re-engineering of a policy, contract provision or settlement that impacts the many can result in accolades and praise of

true proactive leadership. However, when those ideas or pro-
visions go south and do not garner the efficiency or impact
desired, the leader will bear the full brunt of any pushback
by the organization. In fact, sometimes organizations may
second-guess your decisions on other projects based on what
recently did not work out. However, true leaders earn the
respect of an organization despite what may not have worked
out as planned and live to fight another day. That respect
comes with many years of experience, knowledge of how
the organization works, and expertise in one's field.

3. Is there a significant person(s) or experience that you feel helped shape you into the person and leader you are today? If so, please describe.

Unfortunately, I have to say "no." I did not have a mentor;
no one took me under their wing. What I was given was
the opportunity to grow and demonstrate my skill set to
lead. I learned by watching others and always strategizing
what I would do differently if I were in charge and given
the opportunity. The moment came when I was given the
opportunity to take over a unit and to lead the organization
with fresh ideas and a different perspective; to change the
dialogue with the organization's stakeholder and to change
the status quo. As the only Latino executive in HR/Labor
Relations for some time, when given the opportunity to
lead I had to take advantage and be the best at what I did.
I had to lead with authority and expertise in order to gain
the respect of others and the organization as a whole, as
all eyes were watching me and I had to make my mark by
paving the way for other Latinos in my shadow, who are
just waiting for that one opportunity to lead.

4. Describe a challenging event or experience that you would have handled differently, given your present level of knowledge and experience.

(This particular interview answer is very compelling in that it
drives home the challenges faced by new and emergent classes,
a topic that will be explored deeply in later chapters).

All the way back to one's own family culture are deep-seated "rules" of behavior (i.e., how one talks, when one talks, issues of assumed and emergent power). Conversely, there is the outside world's perception of the ethnicity or other cultural identification of an emergent leader. Authority can be challenged in a situation where there are preconceived notions regarding the integrity, abilities, or general fitness to lead. Some of these perceptions are expressed and palpable and others may be on a subconscious level, so the expectation to fail is primed at the pump, so to speak. In reaction to this, a leader from a cultural minority may assume several postures, each with its own social advantages and costs.

Interview #2

1. What do you perceive to be the most important traits or qualities of a good leader? Please explain their significance.

- Know and keep the vision and mission of the profession in the forefront.

I believe that good leaders need to focus on the overall vision of what our profession seeks to do—the positive impact it has for those who have communication disorders, for families, and for the professionals that devote their educational and employment pursuits to these individuals. Organizations have specific missions that should align with this vision; thus, leaders must also serve to carry out those missions effectively.

- Listen and be responsive to administrators, colleagues, and stakeholders.

Effective leaders must be able to receive information and direction from others and communicate information to them effectively. They are often positioned in organizations where they must implement directives from others and be responsible for demonstrating outcomes. They have to know and understand all of their constituents so that they are able to give and get information.

- Use compassion, patience, and humor to relate to others.

Leaders cannot lead effectively unless they are able to make personal and positive connections with others. The goal of leaders is not to make friends or to be liked, but rather to treat everyone with respect and to foster a productive and safe environment of trust and positive interactions. If leaders are in a position to evaluate others regarding performance, they need to support evaluative comments and ratings with evidence.

2. *What are some of the rewards and challenges of being a leader?*

Leading can be a lonely business, so this is one of the challenges. Most leaders in our discipline have a long history of working in the educational or health care systems as SLPs, or in the university setting as faculty members. There are certainly lots of opportunities to demonstrate leadership in these roles. However, when a person assumes a formal role as a leader, the nature of the work can change dramatically. It is often the case that decision-making, reporting, problem-solving, and collecting and holding responsibility for others can create many new challenges. Relationships with colleagues can change also, especially when a leader has responsibilities for managing the time and resources of others.

It is rewarding to lead, especially when the group runs smoothly and outcomes are positive and consistent. It is rewarding to take on challenges and problems and work toward their resolution. The expanded responsibilities of leaders add to their personal and professional growth.

3. *How do you measure or define success as a leader?*

I think the measure of success is the advancement of the vision or mission of the organization and the positive personal and professional development of all involved.

4. How do you deal with internal or external problem-solving?

Problems can be large, small, internal, external, sudden, long-term, and so on. I think leaders deal with problems of one form or another on a daily basis. It is sometimes possible to detect a problem and then create a plan to solve it. At other times, problems must receive immediate attention. The varied nature of problems adds to the stress of being a leader. Problems take time and energy to resolve, so leaders need to be able to prioritize how to use both time and energy to work toward effective solutions.

Personally, I have always tried to deal with problems as quickly and directly as possible. But, I also find that taking a bit of time to make sure I understand the problem is very important, because it reduces the risk of reacting to incomplete information.

5. How do you deal with or prepare for change or facing unknowns?

Change and not knowing what each day will bring is certain, so it is important to have flexibility and confidence.

6. How would you describe your personal leadership style?

My style is to listen to constituents, seek input from others when solving problems and making decisions, provide positive interactions, and share credit for success. I try to be accessible and available for others, even when it reduces the time and focus of getting my own agenda accomplished.

7. Is there a significant person(s) or experience that you feel helped shape you into the person and leader you are today? If so, please describe.

I've had many positive experiences over the course of my 38 years in SLP. Faculty mentors, colleagues, team leaders, co-leaders, specific leadership training, and experience have all shaped my views and my leadership skills and style.

8. What advice would you give to someone in your field who has aspirations of attaining a leadership position?

My advice is to start volunteering for leadership positions at the local level within the individual's sphere of influence. For example, at the student SLP level, being an officer for the local chapter of the National Student Speech-Language-Hearing Association (NSSLHA) is a good place to start. Some state-level associations have student representatives, or students can volunteer to be session monitors at conferences. The best way to start is to get started! Observation of leaders is also important, so that they become role models. Experience is the best way to gain the knowledge and skills required to be a strong leader.

9. Describe a particularly challenging event or experience during which you feel that you overcame obstacles and displayed successful leadership. What was the situation? What made it challenging? What helped you overcome the obstacles?

As chair of a department of communication disorders, I created a task force to allocate and utilize the physical space available to the department members. The space needs were varied and the current space allocations were not balanced to the needs. This was challenging and it required all faculty to work together to determine needs and how the needs could be met given the space available. Open communication created the environment for all to work cooperatively to create a plan and to implement it.

10. Describe a challenging event or experience that you would have handled differently, given your present level of knowledge and experience.

I think it is difficult to know all the factors involved in any given situation and we don't always have the benefit of time when we are trying to make decisions and solve problems. Probably the most challenging time was when an individual sent a personal accusation via email, with a copy to my colleagues. I was stunned, and of course, very upset. I did not respond publicly, but dealt with the matter privately; however, I think my reaction was influenced by emotion. As a leader, I should have taken more time to reflect, get information from the person about their anger, and then respond in a more measured fashion.

Interview #3

1. What do you perceive to be the most important traits or qualities of a good leader? Please explain their significance.

Good leaders are excellent communicators who listen well and take the time to explain information pertinent to their team's success. Such information must include both the positives (what is working) and the negatives (an honest and open look at what needs to be changed). The latter should not result in punishment, but rather reflection on about how to improve in those areas and what resources we need to do so.

Good leaders hire the right team members and are able to evaluate the skills each member can contribute to the team. It is important to allow team members to solve problems and do their assigned work in their own unique style. Allow them to know you are there for guidance and advice but encourage them to develop their own work style. Avoid micromanaging but step in when necessary.

Leading by example is important in terms of ethical and moral decisions. Do what's right, even when cutting corners might be easier. Ask your team to do things that you have tried. Learn to delegate and trust the team's work performance (my biggest challenge). Collaborate to create a collegial work environment and expect others to respect it. When someone is not being collegial, call them on it and remind them they are part of a team. Invite diverse opinions and problem-solving techniques. Encourage faculty to offer their ideas, big and small, and to think out loud to collaborate and create solutions. How can we make it better? What do we need to be more current? Who should we get to speak or teach?

2. What are some of the rewards and challenges of being a leader?

The third interviewee said the rewards of being a leader include having a crackerjack team, watching new faculty come into their own, mentoring professionals, and creating a workplace with an excellent reputation. Challenges mentioned by the interviewee included knowing when to step back, not being afraid to dismiss faculty or employees when they do not perform to expectations, and constantly seeking improvement. He also related that leadership can be a very time consuming job that is also paired with a lot of paperwork, especially during financial difficulty.

3. How do you measure or define success as a leader?

The interviewee said success can be measured in terms of (1) outcomes, (2) program data, (3) feedback from surveys by both students and faculty members, (4) whether alumni are willing to work with or supervise students from their alma mater, and (5) long-term faculty.

4. How do you deal with internal or external problem-solving?

Generally by facing things head on with the truth as I know it. It makes it easier.

5. How do you deal with or prepare for change or facing unknowns?

The interviewee stated the importance of utilizing research and data analytics, which can support an objective argument for a course of action. Soliciting advice from colleagues and peers or forming focus groups can also be beneficial. Lastly, attending professional conferences at the state and national level helps leaders stay informed about current practices and education.

6. How would you describe your personal leadership style?

The interviewee described himself as a collaborative leader with adroit communication skills, who is both organized and honest. He is decisive in a manner that allows time to process information before making a decision, but also has a sense of humor and support from his faculty. He endorses celebrating as a group for accomplishments, birthdays, and even promotions.

7. Is there a significant person(s) or experience who you feel helped shape you into the person and leader you are today? If so, please describe.

I am one of ten children who often organized plays, games, and fundraisers. My teachers would often put me in charge of class activities and I enjoyed the challenge. In my first professional job, I saw there were some people on my team who were slacking off and not doing their job. With another co-worker we developed a program and engaged our entire team in determining how best to run the program and gave them the freedom to choose what areas of the program they wanted to participate in. Then we divided the grunt work among us. Eventually we wrote up a description of the program and submitted it to a peer reviewed journal; I published my first article at age 27.

8. What advice would you give to someone in your field who has aspirations of attaining a leadership position?

Be loyal to your team, communicate the parts they need to know to get their jobs done, and be positive even when negative thoughts abound.

9. Describe a particularly challenging event or experience during which you feel that you overcame obstacles and displayed successful leadership. What was the situation? What made it challenging? What helped you overcome the obstacles?

The interviewee related that the probation period from the Council on Academic Accreditation was humiliating. He navigated through this difficult period by reaching out for support from both the students and faculty, and asking for help. He also stood up for himself and demanded from himself a higher quality of progress and growth in confidence. This confidence allowed him to effectively delegate while moving up the leadership hierarchy to his goal.

10. Describe a challenging event or experience that you would have handled differently, given your present level of knowledge and experience.

Hiring a faculty member I knew wasn't going to fit in and was inexperienced simply because we didn't want to lose the faculty line. Most likely the college would not have allowed me to hire the following year. Required so much training, mentoring, and still didn't work out. Trust your gut.

Interview #4

1. What do you perceive to be the most important traits or qualities of a good leader? Please explain their significance.

- Assessment—the ability to look at overall conditions, capabilities of personnel, and parameters of projects at hand.
- Team development—the leader will only be as strong as his weakest link.
- Thinking outside the box—the ability to offer multiple solutions to problems.

2. What are some of the rewards and challenges of being a leader?

Rewards are achieving goals and personal satisfaction. Leaders want to be positive achievers and recognized. The challenge [of being a leader] is possible failure [and] unknown intervening factors.

3. *How do you measure or define success as a leader?*

Measurements include establishing benchmarks, completing goals, setting dates for deliverables, and self-monitoring. Good leaders know when they need to get extra resources.

4. *How do you deal with internal or external problem-solving?*

Define the problem, get necessary resources and staff, know costs and time frames to solve the problem.

5. *How do you deal with or prepare for change or facing unknowns?*

Look for opportunities to "pre-view" based on experiences of others; adjust to the unknown and seek assistance for unexpected developments.

6. *How would you describe your personal leadership style?*

I try to be supportive and get input, but am aware of [my own] responsibility for the big decisions as the leader. People should have book smarts as well as day-to-day life experience. Opportunities to be independent force you to engage and manage better.

7. *What advice would you give to someone in your field who has aspirations of attaining a leadership position?*

Complete as much study in your topic area as possible. Network!!

8. *Describe a particularly challenging event or experience during which you feel that you overcame obstacles and displayed successful leadership. What was the situation? What made it challenging? What helped you overcome the obstacles?*

Most challenging was a failed project, but because of strong prior relationships, I was able to get a good short-term solution in place until a long-term plan could be established.

9. Describe a challenging event or experience that you would have handled differently, given your present level of knowledge and experience.

In hiring, it is hard to predict how a candidate will work out; develop a more detailed interviewing process to avoid [problems] in the future!

Interview Summary

At the core of these interviews, the most frequently mentioned features of an effective leader were vision, evaluation, and communication. All interviewees conveyed a need for leaders to demonstrate adroit analysis and assessment skills in some capacity —especially when choosing faculty members. Additionally, clear communication with team members about the overall goals and the tasks of each individual was cited as an imperative skill for leaders. Leaders must use their communication skills to develop effective team members and faculty during the planning and organization phase of any long-term goal. Lastly, decision-making was discussed. Being a top-notch leader requires having the decision-making skills to focus on and facilitate the achievement of long-term goals. Decision-making includes interpreting information from, and perspectives of others, assessing the needs of clients and the organization, and implementing a course of action conducive to those goals and needs.

Harvard Business Review Models

The competencies outlined by the above interviewees can be compared to those recently collected by the *Harvard Business Review* in a survey of 195 leaders in 15 countries over 30 global organizations (Giles, 2016). The competencies identified by the *Harvard Business Review* are summarized below:

The importance of setting and sticking to high standards is that it ensures that the workplace remains a safe and trusting environment for everyone (Giles, 2016). The ability to self-organize results in employees and staff members who feel more empowered, and consequently, act in a more productive and proactive manner than their counterparts (Giles, 2016). Fostering connection can also impact the productivity and emotional well-being of employees and staff members, by boosting morale and encouraging positivity and feelings of support and encouragement. Lastly, nurturing growth and learning presents opportunities for an open exchange of ideas, which ensures that everyone's thoughts and ideas are heard and makes everyone feel that they are an integral member of the team as a whole. Nurturing growth reflects a leader's recognition that the success of the organization depends on everyone contributing and working collaboratively toward a common goal, rather than limiting themselves to a very narrow scope and vision, which could ultimately work against the organization instead of enabling them to thrive. Thus, the majority of the competencies cited by the interviewees coincide with those specified by the *Harvard Business Review*. The overlap in qualities and competencies viewed as signs of effective leadership demonstrates that some leadership skills may be considered universal.

Conclusion

Exhaustive searches of literature did not show many recent studies about leadership qualities. This may be due to both the interdisciplinary nature of the topic and methodological constraints (e.g., inability to match subject entities). A case study approach may be useful in the future.

There are however, several resources currently available for novice and seasoned leaders alike that may be helpful, particularly for SLPs looking to attain leadership positions in the near future or to further develop their leadership skills in specific areas. For instance, institutions such as Atlas (Academic Training, Leadership, & Assessment Services; http://www.atlasleadership.com/home.html) offer training programs and workshops and seminars in academic leadership, as well as publications on leadership and leadership assessment tools (see references for further information).

For current and upcoming leaders in speech-pathology, ASHA offers a Leadership Development Program (http://www.asha .org/about/governance/leadership-development-program/). The program consists of a year-long training course that includes workshops, webinars, the opportunity to volunteer, and participation in a leadership project (see references to obtain further information). Both of these programs offer great potential opportunities for novice and seasoned leaders alike.

Trending

In Chapter 3, we explore organizations in which SLP leaders may practice and/or be cultivated.

Reflection

Which leadership qualities do you think are the most important? Which leadership qualities have you observed in those around you? What are the relative strengths and weaknesses of each quality?

References

Carozza, L. (2010). *Science of successful supervision and mentorship.* San Diego, CA: Plural.

Fine, D. J. (2002). Establishing competencies for healthcare managers. *Healthcare Executive, 17*(2), 66–67.

Gardner, H. (1999). Multiple approaches to understanding. In C. M. Reigeluth (Ed.), Instructional design theories and models: *A new paradigm of instructional theory* (Vol. 2, pp. 69–89). Mahwah, NJ: Lawrence Erlbaum.

Giles, S. (2016). *The most important leadership competencies, according to leaders around the world.* Retrieved from https://hbr.org/2016/03/the-most-important-leadershipcompetencies-according-to-leaders-around-the-world

Goleman, D. (2004). *What makes a leader?* Retrieved from https://hbr.org/2004/01/what-makes a-leader

Hartman, S., & Crow, S. (2002). Executive development in healthcare during times of turbulence: Top management perceptions and recommendations. *Journal of Management in Medicine, 16*(4–5), 359–370. https://doi.org/10.1108/02689230210446535

Pilling, S., & Slattery, J. (2004). Management competencies: Intrinsic or acquired? What competencies are required to move into speech-pathology management and beyond? *Australian Health Review, 27*(1), 84–92. https://doi.org/10.1071/AH042710084

Rao, P. (2006). Emotional intelligence: The sine qua non for a clinical leadership toolbox. *Journal of Communication Disorders, 39*(4), 310–319. https://doi.org/10.1016/j.jcomdis.2006.02.006

Additional Resources

Cole, P. R. (1987). Attaining positions of leadership. *ASHA, 29*(12), 23–25. Retrieved from https://www.ncbi.nlm.nih.gov/pubmed/3322292

Moore, S. M. (1993). Teams and teamwork. Reflections on leadership. *ASHA, 35*(6–7), 47–48. Retrieved from https://www.ncbi.nlm.nih.gov/pubmed/8216466

Rizzo, S. (1994). Graduate programs fall short. *ASHA, 36*(11), 65–66. Retrieved from http://mbbsdost.com/Graduate-programs-fall-short-ASHA-Rizzo-SR--1994 Nov/pubmed/10813981

3

Organizations in Which Speech-Language Pathologists May Participate in Leadership Positions

Linda S. Carozza

Put yourself where your strengths can produce results.
—Peter F. Drucker, Harvard Business Review

Learning Objective

- Readers will learn about opportunities in which leadership may emerge. Some of these opportunities may be pre-existing, in an evolutionary stage, or can be developed as needs of an organization mature.

Think Question

What are some potential benefits for an SLP in taking on a leadership role within an organization?

Background

Institutions may be formal or informal. A simple team meeting may be the start of a career in leadership when a new clinician observes the qualities of a designated leader and other dynamics that support or oppose leadership. Opportunities for leadership abound and recognizing and capitalizing on such moments are integral for any developing leader.

Some of this material comes from the literature outside of the training of a licensed practitioner; therefore, this chapter is aimed at sharpening the lens of leadership both in smaller entities and in larger, regulated entities, from the standpoint of collecting public monies and related accountabilities.

Organizational Culture

First and foremost, it is critical for young leaders to learn the defined culture of organizations in which they participate. This may come in the form of a new-manager orientation or a distributed table of the organizational structure and a policy and procedures manual.

Entering a leadership position in established environments is a high-challenge task, which requires both experience and acumen. The set of expected accomplishments and agendas is important to grasp initially so that managers do not get mired down in navigating the culture first, and can instead hit the ground running. However, also having knowledge of the specific culture, subculture, and internal structure is critical to surviving and thriving in the organization. The internal structure may be visible or not so visible, and insight into the power dynamics and decision-making tree may take time to develop. Thus, pre-existing knowledge of the stated vision, mission, and mandates of the organization is highly important. Along with this comes the concept of what the deliverables are and how progress is measured. In addition to the overall organization's deliverables are a manager's own deliverables, which generally include adding expertise, insight, and inspiration for how things can be done more influentially and effectively.

Organizational Setting

Another variable that new managers must be concerned with is the setting in which the organization exists. Settings can range from small, discreet operations, such as a solo private practice, an outpatient clinic, or a small organization that requires a new budget and expansion, to larger settings with concurrent accountabilities to clients, families, allied interprofessional communities, a board of trustees, or other oversight group. The overarching interest of the program leader is always to ensure the common good with as much input as possible from varied voices so that internal, external, and growth agendas may be addressed. If managers are adept at engaging and guiding people, they may be able to draw on a vast amount of skill and cooperation. If not, they may find themselves working alone and frustratingly reinventing the wheel.

Current Leadership Program Offerings

A great start to a career in management is student exposure to leadership while in graduate school via coursework or student organizations, such as the NSSLHA. ASHA also provides many opportunities for growth including formal leadership programs. By taking advantage of training opportunities, prospective managers can learn about the intricacies of advisory boards and other constituencies that have influence over the services provided to a given population, whether the population is a student body or a patient caseload. Careful study avoids a sink or swim attitude that was prevalent in past years when people were expected to learn on the job rather than come in with specific skill sets. It is vital for clinicians to handle their managerial roles in much the same way they would manage a practice—that is, by having guidelines and overarching policies in place and to avoid judging situations on a case-by-case basis, which can lead to uneven application of policies and even potentially expose novice managers to complaints of discrimination and bias.

According to University of Cincinnati (UC) Health News (Cosse, 2009), leadership roles may even elevate speech pathologists to influential positions responsible for new policy development or for guiding educational strategies and funding. In that article, Cosse outlines how Dr. Nancy Creaghead marshaled resources at UC to train doctoral students to pursue leadership roles in addition to their work in educational research. Dr. Creaghead indicated that students who work with leaders are more able to move into positions of authority. Overall, the goal of training advanced faculty—those who can go beyond the classroom and lead policy and innovation—will be a driving force in the profession's advancement.

Advancing Speech-Language Pathology Assistant Leadership

As more than half (roughly 52%) of SLPs work in educational settings (ASHA, 2017), it is critical to understand the hierarchy of decision makers in your professional setting. Readings outside of the professional, clinical domain of speech pathology are critical towards understanding where leadership opportunities for SLPs may be found, and open courseware, such as the Organizational Leadership and Change course offered via MIT is free and informative for emergent leaders (Klein, 2009). That course describes its goals as focusing "on practical experience that blends theory and practice. Students reflect on prior leadership experiences and then apply lessons learned to further develop their leadership capabilities" (Course Description, https://ocw.mit.edu/courses/sloan-school-of-management/15-317-organizational-leadership-and-change-summer-2009/). The course requires active participation and has assigned deliverables. Students can design their own course objectives to answer managerial concerns relevant to meeting the responsibilities in a new environment with both crossover skills and insight gained from the course, furthering self-growth. This would be advantageous for managers engaged in writing a strategic plan for an organization, or tasked with developing or serving on an advisory board in a health or educational setting. The task may change, but the requisite skills of delegating, following through, team building, and sustained communication cross over into many aspects of organizational growth and change. Many forward-thinking organizations invest in developing these skills, helping to keep their focus on meeting the everchanging needs of consumers and advisors.

Established graduate programs exist for the many SLPs who find themselves in school leadership roles. A chief example is the Harvard University master's program in School Leadership (Harvard University, 2017). Experienced professionals across a range of fields gather to learn to deal with the challenges of non-profit, for-profit, philanthropic, and other entities. The program can benefit professionals who want to launch their own private schools or educational programs and need the well-rounded education that allows them to promote and gain support for forward-thinking initiatives. According to the programs description, candidates learn to lead people, lead schools and organizations, and lead learning (Harvard University, 2017).

Dr. Nancy Swigert attests that as of 2007, only 10.7% of ASHA certified SLPs reported an administrative role as their primary function (Swigert, 2008). She wrote that "when you subtract the 0.4% who chair an educational or research program, we are left with 10.3% who work in an administrative role, and we don't know how many of those are in health care (p. 22)." This small percentage is extremely important because it could reflect a lack of leadership opportunities for SLPs due to a lack of sufficient managerial training during their education. In contrast, other health professions such as nursing have access to career ladders that facilitate development of management skills. A study by Benner (1984) describes the levels of expertise in nursing from novice to expert, based on experiential learning. Nursing training includes learning how to recognize excellence in leadership, how to encourage professional development, and how to facilitate career advancement. Advancement in nursing, in fact, may depend more on learning leadership than clinical techniques, which is a vast difference from SLP continuing education sequences, which focus on maintaining core competencies for bedside or in-school service delivery.

Guilford, Graham, and Scheuerle (2006), stress the need for clinical skill development and management training for SLPs wanting to pursue administrative, as opposed to clinical positions. A worthy goal is for more SLPs to take advantage of formal management training in both health care and educational service delivery settings, to have the flexibility of choice, and to have a voice in their practice setting. This would grow the number of SLP professionals leadership positions with the promise of succession by like-minded and well-trained individuals.

ASHA encourages the talented and aspiring leaders of tomorrow by providing opportunities for leadership in special interest groups, committees, state organizations, and many other roles. SLPs have an opportunity draw on the experience of others to influence the profession's future.

The featured article in the *The ASHA Leader* newsletter (Law, 2015) spoke to this point. It focused on SLPs and speech scientists who bring their knowledge and expertise to positions creating change in corporations, research funding agencies, university systems, and all levels of government. The professionals interviewed in the article bring great insight into the peripheries of leadership. Many echoed the idea that leadership skills are akin to skills already needed for careers in speech-language pathology and related professions. Former ASHA leader Tommie Robinson Jr. states, "there is something about our skill set . . . that's inherently related to [those positions]" (Law, 2015). As professional facilitators of communication, SLPs can mold their experiences into qualities that fit leadership roles.

Several interviewees mentioned early involvement in committees or boards as kickstarting their journey into management. These roles were available at professional organizations and organizations both related to and completely outside of the interviewees' professions. Notably, the leaders who discussed their paths all strayed away from the career ladder model of progression. Instead, many found leadership roles by jumping in from different areas. Whether they moved into SLP from another profession or changed from a clinical setting to a government or business setting, many paths do not follow a linear pattern; instead, they more closely follow Sheryl Sandberg's jungle gym model (Jacobs, 2013).

Another common theme mentioned among the interviews was a sense of reward from helping others, even when tasks may not have directly affected patients or clients. Although leadership usually entails a level of public visibility, some positions require less action in the public eye. Leadership for many interviewees, including Colonels Tuten and Cooper, manifested in the form of mentorship. Cooper mentions, "our growth as leaders also comes in taking responsibility for making sure our profession will have a next generation—and there are many levels to do that through the research lab, clinic, classroom, or hospital" (Law, 2015, p. 58). This statement was true even for many of the interviewees who moved past traditional SLP occupations into government and military positions.

Law (2015) also profiles several prominent leaders who received CSD degrees but went beyond the scope of clinical practice to take on leadership roles in related fields. Some of the individuals profiled include Tommie Robinson, former ASHA president; Michelle Garcia, founder of the highly acclaimed Social Thinking program; and Barry Prizant, co-founder of the Social Communication, Emotional Regulation, and Transactional Support (SCERTS) model, among others. Some of these individuals described themselves as having leadership qualities from an early age—thus, taking on a leadership role was a natural progression in their careers—whereas others never saw themselves as leaders and took on their roles as a means of pursuing their passions. Some cited seeking to fill a void or gap within a specific organization, or tackling a larger social or legislative issue plaguing a certain group of individuals affected by a hearing or communication disorder as an impetus.

Although the paths taken to their current roles differed significantly, all of these influential individuals agreed that it was well worth the risks and challenges encountered, and that they learned invaluable lessons along the way. According to Colonel Tuten, she learned that qualities that make a great leader include, "ownership of mistakes, willingness to mentor, vulnerability, and a staff that complements the leader's strengths and weaknesses" (Law, 2015, p. 58). Michelle Garcia also brought up the importance of being open-minded and having a broad perspective; she described her journey by stating that, "everything informed the next stage, and I don't think I could have developed this at all if I were sitting in a bubble, having one paradigm and one view of the world" (Law, 2015, p. 51).

Reflection

In what ways can you envision leadership opportunities emerging? What circumstances call for trained leaders and which may be opportunities for leadership to develop?

References

American Speech-Language-Hearing Association. (2017). *Supply and demand resource list for speech-language pathologists.* Retrieved from http://www.asha.org/uploadedFiles/Supply-Demand-SLP.pdf

Benner, P. (1984). *From novice to expert: Excellence and power in clinical nursing practice.* Menlo Park, CA: Addison-Wesley.

Cosse, K. (2009, November). *Leadership roles might hold key to attract speech language pathologist educators.* Retrieved from http://health news.uc.edu/publications/findings/?/9446/9460/

Good Reads. (2017). Harvard Business School press quotes. Retrieved from https://www.goodreads.com/author/quotes/2244.Harvard_Business_School_Press

Guilford, A., Graham, S. J., & Scheuerle, J. (2006). *The speech-language pathologist: From novice to expert.* Boston, MA: Allyn & Bacon.

Harvard University. (2017). School leadership. Retrieved from https://www.gse.harvard.edu/masters/slp

Jacobs, D. L. (2013, March 14). Why a career jungle gym is better than a career ladder. *Forbes.* Retrieved from https://www.forbes.com/sites/deborahljacobs/2013/03/14/why-a-careerjungle-gym-is-better-than-a-career-ladder/#11fabc4e1248

Klein, J. (2009) *Organizational leadership and change.* Massachusetts Institute of Technology. Retrieved from https://ocw.mit.edu

Law, B. M. (2015, November). The beat of a different leader. *The ASHA Leader, 20*(11), 46–61. https://doi.org/10.1044/leader.FTR3.2011 2015.46

Swigert, N. B. (2008, November). Management roles for speech-language pathologists in health care. *The ASHA Leader, 13*(16), 22–24. https://doi.org/10.1044/leader.FTR6.13162008.22

4

Starting Point for Leadership

Linda S. Carozza

A natural leader in speech-language pathology is one who appreciates the depth and breadth of the profession. The privilege of leading and training professionals to learn and carry on this work starts with this recognition.

—Linda S. Carozza

Learning Objectives

- To describe leadership maturation from the standpoint of how to acquire the depth of experience that allows one to attain a personal and unique sense of mission and vision.
- To understand concepts related to leadership essentials, including the importance of both seasoned mentoring professionals and the support of a team in establishing a leadership career. For the purposes of this chapter only, leadership and management are equated and used interchangeably.

Introduction

Leadership starts with self-knowledge. The old adage that "there is no I in team" sparks the incentive to study organizational team building; however, leaders must know themselves very well before taking a place on a team. Leaders who don't recognize the importance of self-knowledge until already in a leadership position find themselves in a quandary when projects stagnate or staff engage in behaviors that are resistant to overall program goals. Self-knowledge can be gained numerous ways, from previous life or work experience to ongoing corporate coaching or self-improvement instruction, and it is most beneficial when acquired prior to taking on senior management roles. This is especially important in today's fast-paced markets, where managers may move between organizations and need to work simultaneously on varied programs, affecting outcomes, morale, and service delivery expectations, and with accountability to multiple factions.

The Importance of Self-Assessment and Self-Knowledge

Leaders who are nuanced, fluid, and self-aware in their pursuit of goals have many advantages over managers who seek outcomes solely by measurable standards of performance. Although this may seem like an improbable point of view, consider that sustainability of an organization over time and performance metrics (such as number of visits by governing boards or enrollees) do not tell the whole story of a program's efficiency. It is essential that a leader know the pulse of their units. The pulse takes the shape of the energy of performers within a department, along with levels of engagement and overall job satisfaction among the employees. Certain leaders, especially new-to-the-job leaders, will assume a certain lack of accountability for team members' prior working patterns and make a decision to let teams settle in after a managerial transition. This position has merits in that it allows leaders to best make extremely strategic observations about a department's long-term prospects during this transitional period. The scope of these observations should include overall strengths and weaknesses, employee buy-in and motivation and interpersonal and intrapersonal relationships. This list is not exhaustive, as an effective leader may not know what situations are observationally important until they experience them, particularly in the rapidly changing educational and health industry landscapes.

When leaders succumb to achievement criteria that do not consider *both* qualitative and quantitative measurements together, they are missing half of a program's potential. Without a combination of measures of success, a leader may not be able to assess properly a program or decision due to a simple lack of exposure to information. Leaders must have an overall vision and specific strategic skills to achieve said vision, such as the ability to set goals and priorities and to optimize resource utilization. However, it is harder, yet just as important, to define the leader's own self-knowledge. Self-knowledge leads to a more empathetic and nurturing leadership style; one that is not focused solely on deliverables and making the numbers. Leaders who manage solely from the head and have no heart in their management style may not effectively capitalize on long-term growth and potential of an established unit, especially one that runs on momentum gained from knowing and applying their strengths and weaknesses to correct issues and achieve goals.

How is self-knowledge gained while working on intense project management with high-level and talented employees who have the same high expectations of their leader? Self-knowledge is very ephemeral and is an ongoing process of awareness and maturity. Young leaders are very different in their use of strategies and resources than they will be in later life when experiences and maturity will have imparted knowledge transferable to the workplace. So, novice leaders must increase their knowledge of viable techniques for cultivating self-awareness, especially in the workplace. Any supervisor, manager or other individual with authority to make decisions that alter the workplace—regardless of novice or advanced status—are similarly affected. Any such person of authority may find subordinates or co-workers who are not ready to engage in self-growth practices, and thus, leadership can be lonely, even for those with the intention of growth and compassion.

Steps to self-growth for leaders start with taking time away from the technical components of daily departmental business to think about who they are and what they value. Self-growth is a very complicated process. Colleagues may express opinions about different resources to enhance the process of gaining self-knowledge (including peer-groups, on-the-job retreats, taking independent coursework, or even engaging in psychotherapeutic counseling). Regardless of method, the goal is to examine feelings, thoughts, and emotions experienced on the job in reaction to task demands, personalities, and scenarios that occur. As human beings, we desire good relationships along with good results. This goes for leaders and staff. Self-growth is inherently difficult to measure, and is diametrically different from the performance management tools and spreadsheets taught in business schools. Although there is a definite need to speak the language of an industry using clear and concise achievement measurements (such as year-end performance reviews), wise managers know there is a more nuanced underlying thread for how the workforce will best achieve its goals.

New leaders will confront the relevance of self-awareness while initially on the job or sometimes as a by-product when projects derail, or tension and dissension are the flavor of the day at departmental meetings, or when there is more collateral communication than frank and respectful interaction during meetings. Managers who are insecure in their position come across as not being authentic and this quickly erodes group effort as well as managers' morale. Therefore, leaders must make efforts to increase self-knowledge of personality, style, reaction behaviors, communication techniques, and all the subtle signals that convey a sense of departmental cohesion and organization to staff members. No one can function well without a certain sense of personal and emotional safety. Providing a common safety net for group members is essential, although a caveat here is that managers are not expected to manage major or significant personality disorders requiring additional resources, which is beyond the scope of this discussion. Secure managers can recognize common interpersonal miscommunications and react confidently to both routine and escalating problems.

Therefore, leader designees bring a certain sense of self-knowledge to their job, with answers to questions such as, how am I seen? How do I wish to be seen? How do I respond during interpersonal office communications? With subordinates? With peers? With higher-level management? What has been effective for me? What has not?. Many leaders have idealized goals of what makes a perfect manager; but in reality, managers must be who they are, and they will vary on what makes each a strong, yet effective and compassionate leader. This individuality can sometimes cause conflict in environments that have a different culture than the one in which a manager is used to performing. Knowing oneself, others, and the operating environment are three prongs of business leadership success. Learning the answers to the types of self-knowledge questions just posed can be achieved in many ways. For example, there may be an informal group for socialization, a walk around the various offices, or formal mentorship in certain environments. There is also the matter of seen versus unseen elements; the official culture may be different than the culture that workers perceive. This adds an additional layer of responsibility to a manager, one that may not be reflected in quantitative performance reviews. Integrating a genuine interest in self-growth, establishing or re-establishing communications with staff and significant peers, as well as being a keen observer in workplace mores is key to leadership success. There are managers who do well because cooperation and cohesion in a unit may allow them to outperform those who continually watch the bottom-line for compliance and productivity. The insightful senior manager is one who recognizes growing leaders so that organizations can retain key professionals and mature accordingly, rather than stopping and starting new agendas over and over again whenever there is a turnover of leaders who never establish themselves or the department's cohesion. There will sometimes be dissension or stalemates; however, the leader who approaches their position with an appreciation of the human variables within both themselves and other key players is way ahead of the game.

Nurturing Self-Awareness

In the *Harvard Business Review*, Hougaard, Carter, and Afton (2018) describe very precisely how leaders can nurture qualities of self-awareness. All leaders in different disciplines can benefit from the techniques described. Some techniques suggested are centered around mindfulness, and include taking work breaks throughout the day and paying attention to the environment. Environmental awareness includes listening to what is being said, how it is said and in what context, and how communication(s) are received. Modeling oneself after an established successful leader is another strategy that can be helpful. Striving to know oneself brings peace of mind to the myriad tasks and ambiguities decision makers are faced with. Leadership focused on maturity and intricate problem-solving, rather than just task achievement alone, leads to overall satisfaction and a department able to handle both routine and unanticipated work challenges more smoothly.

Peripheral Skills, Expertise, and Qualities Essential to Leadership

This brings us to another question: Can someone be a great leader without technical expertise? A strong industry background and up-to-date skills are necessary for staff motivation. Knowledge of the technical aspect of health or educational standards on national and international horizons is indeed a formidable expertise to bring to the work environment. As effective communication is so closely linked with technological advances now (i.e., increase in digital and virtual presentations, videoconferencing, etc.), both flexibility in learning and a global perspective are required. Few young leaders know the global landscape and have a long view of specialization that the fast growth world we live in demands. Leaders must also demonstrate an ability to motivate curiosity and ambition in their staff, and have highly precise oral and written communication skills (especially important in a field with communication in the title). Subordinates may be overly analytical or critical of their leader's communication skills as they are (generally) professional teachers or service providers. The ability to create is vastly different than the ability to edit and critique, and, forearmed with this knowledge, effective leaders ensure that communication is extremely clear in content and context. Additional skills that leaders must demonstrate are critical thinking and effective problem-solving for workplace challenges, which are essential for managing outcomes and expectations in an organization. Short-term problem-solving is different from providing longer term solutions, which aim at understanding and preventing recurrent issues by analyzing previous contributions, mitigating circumstances, and other variables.

Other critical skills beyond domain expertise are the abilities to identify work teams, delegate, and supervise projects to completion. Leaders must be able to deal with a vast quantity of information, understand core group dynamics, and distribute meaningful work products to their team.

Only having skill in one area, that is, of communications and its pathologies, is therefore insufficient to tackle management goals. Leaders, through commitment to a vision and mission, inspire professional trust among the employees sufficient that all can satisfactorily work towards common goals. What are the requisite skills and how can leaders ensure that they have them all to navigate each stage of managerial evolution? Good communicating, the ability to ask for help, leading through example, and more precise performance markers for the team is vital.

What happens when life happens? It is inevitable that leaders will experience life situations that call them away from the workplace. This can be traumatic for the manager at times in small or startup operations, where managers function akin to sole proprietors. Being a manager may mean tasks are difficult to delegate, yet leaders must stop and think about the solutions they would recommend to subordinates impacted by a personal event that pulls them away. The first thing leaders in this situation must do is analyze available resources, then consider the pros and cons of self-disclosure in the organization. There may be different possible levels of accommodations and inevitably, even managers must recognize their own humanity. Therefore, short-term limited schedules, distributing workload, or family medical leave are all options. It is difficult to contemplate, but wise organizations and managers prepare for future unknowns to protect their work products. Preparations must be made, keeping the most valuable resource in mind; that is, human capital. The concerns of institutional stakeholders must be considered, as must the needs of the manager whose return to work may be considered more valuable than a break in service.

Leaders in the health or educational service industry are first and foremost communicators. Communication can be thought of as making information common to all. In order to effectively communicate, leaders must first gain awareness of their own communication skills and limitations, through directed self-study. Having a combination of intuitive "smarts" (sometimes called people smarts) and technical smarts (sometimes called work smarts), and having the ability to recognize their own human limitations are also important. Additionally, because no man is an island, smart leaders know to look forward and back on the career ladder; to recognize the importance of individuals who mentored them in the past and typically, to go on to mentor junior professionals in the future.

Importance of Mentorship

The significance of mentorship cannot be overlooked in a discussion of emergent leadership. Although most authors would agree that knowledge can be attained through advanced certificate training, the practicalities of a specific setting may be such that an external ear is also be necessary.

According to Pilling and Slattery (2004), an area of expertise that most new leaders report feeling uncomfortable with is finance. This can be a complicated competency for which to seek mentorship, as internal circumstances determine how an institution establishes and modifies financial planning. Internal circumstances could include a lack of interdepartmental communication or limited access to finance professionals within the organization. There are benefits, then, to seeking alliances with groups of business professionals outside of the workplace, such as those who started their own businesses. Independent business owners would be know how to establish and monitor a business plan, and would understand growth and marketing. As departments are sometimes based on a bottom-line business model in today's economy, consultation on the demographics, need, competition, trends, and general analysis of various departments is often valuable for planning.

In practice, most leadership professionals have been mentored or have at least observed the pros and cons of their own supervisors in the past. This is, in a sense, a form of reverse mentorship; you get to see what is undesirable, as well as what is admirable, in a given leadership style. Most transitional leaders would be wise to seek a multitiered approach to honing their skills. This would involve using the existing shared competencies that emerge from being a senior professional in a discipline-specific domain (such as speech-language pathology), and identifying additional competencies that are required but were not part of one's initial education. There are numerous opportunities to attend business seminars, join business groups, and earn advanced certificates in budgeting, project management, dealing with conflict, team building, and other skills. Participating in training helps strengthen new leaders' intellectual preparedness and provides an external forum for issues that inevitably arise.

Career planning should take into account that people may be inherently better suited to one job environment than another, so professionals should not lose faith if an initial experience with leadership is less than rewarding. Experiences, both good and bad, comprise a path of self-discovery and maturity in a career, and everyone experiences bumps in the road. There are open settings that cultivate an authentic, nurturing atmosphere, and others where differences in opinions and ideas are less valued. To decode the priorities of a given environment, it is necessary to observe and understand the management style of the chief administrator.

One way to grasp the style of upper management is to read about their work and what advice they have passed on to formative leaders. A flexible style that can adapt to the voices of a new generation of professionals has broad appeal, especially given today's culturally diverse and multigenerational community served, that is, the new generation of professionals. An effective mentor would have the ability to actively listen without judgment. Cultivating this ability involves the same characteristics described in counselors; such as reflecting back what was said, affirming others' values, seeking compromise, and a willingness to retain commitment.

For mentoring purposes, some senior leaders establish formal collaborative leadership trainings, so that new leaders gain confidence and work together more securely. Feldman (2018) describes an extensive tiered model of leadership development. She comments on the avoidance of *groupthink*, defined as "a pattern of thought characterized by self-deception, forced manufacture of consent, and conformity to group values and ethics" (https://www.merriam-webster.com/dictionary/groupthink), which is antithetical to the notion of building a team where each member contributes according to their own strengths. Feldman gives specific examples of how to nurture leadership teams and imbue individuals with a sense of power so they can develop self-confidence and sustain leadership.

In order to achieve team-building, group interaction not directly related to specific organizational issues are needed. This can be accomplished via arranged retreats, in which there are joint readings, analyses of new material, and opportunities for self-assessment. Retreats can lead to renewed vigor for workplace demands, brought about by deepening networks of mutual trust and greater confidence in any or all individual(s) on a team. The style of and approach to planned outside development activities can differ, and it is a unique organization overall that fosters the development of leaders from within in this manner. Therefore, it would behoove new leaders and those who mentor leaders (i.e., upper level management) to research other institutions or organizations who take this approach to team-building. Unfortunately, in the health or education sectors (non-profit), it is not always common to have the budget that affords this type of training. However, in corporate or for-profit settings, management development is a career-long process and systematic trainings are part of the career ladder. Training in effective communication relates back in many ways to the speech-language pathology background and is paramount to group performance. Clinicians with corporate experience have potentially been exposed to the differing training styles in non-profit and for-profit enterprises, and thusly may have more insight than those without this experience.

Recognizing a need, professional organizations, ASHA chief among them, have developed unique training initiatives for emergent leaders. These include leadership institutes, conventions, special-interest-group activities, and other forthcoming ventures described elsewhere in this book. Emergent leaders must be committed to self-development, and a stable home life and firmly set career expectations are important to achieving this goal. In fact, the notion of setting career expectations may be the secret sauce in the equation. Career change and transition sometimes occur not because of failed competencies or potential, but because professionals are increasingly expected to successfully mitigate challenges not commonly faced by previous generations of leaders. In effect, growth happens the hard way unless specific programs focusing on mitigating and meeting the changing needs of any profession (such as ASHA's Student to Empowered Professional Mentoring Program [S.T.E.P.] for young career professionals) are utilized.

Mentorships can be continually developed throughout one's professional career, and one's suitability for the role of both mentor and mentee is a significant area of academic research (Carozza, 2010). Mentorship is a mechanism for recruiting and retaining the most talented of the next generation of professionals, who in turn become future leaders. The mentor to mentee "watch one, do one, teach one" approach produces gifted mentors working with an engaged and informed future leader.

I encourage a broad perspective in thinking about mentoring relationships and communications between junior and senior level employees, with a goal of overall organizational growth. Our profession has developed many perspectives on being a reflective practitioner, and adapting them to become both a reflective mentor and mentee is highly encouraged. At the same time, mentor/mentee pairings are individually unique, and one perspective may not fit all situations. In much the same way that the allied health professions learn from related disciplines, such as nursing, physical therapy, occupational therapy and psychiatric medicine, it behooves speech-language pathologists to take an interdisciplinary approach to mentorship. Identifying, building, and sustaining new and emergent leaders is a long-term part of strategic growth in any organization. The path to leadership has many starting points and intersections along the journey. Feldman (2018) posits that developing effective leadership teams is important to the success of any organization, regardless of that organization's size. She also affirms that investing in the social capital of an organization is a building block to organizational growth and integrity to move forward.

The Role of the Team

The ideals of leadership involve principles of psychology and organizational theory, which many communication professionals may not have studied from the standpoint of applying those principles to leading their own organizations. Despite knowledge of interpersonal and intercultural communication, many senior professionals in speech-language pathology study these topics as they relate to others, not to themselves. This is ironic in that senior SLPs may consult and offer their services as communication specialists to other businesses, but may never have had the opportunity to turn this particular lens on themselves. It becomes a real challenge for SLPs to confidently believe in their own abilities to manage the communication of others without this self-reflection.

In a quest to learn and convey overarching psychology and business principles that I have uncovered during the process of becoming a leader, I have engaged in many self-improvement exercises and professional programs to enhance my knowledge. So much of what we do in the office setting is learned and honed earlier in life through childhood or early work dynamics and finding the motivation to change ourselves and direct change in others may be more difficult later in life. I embrace the work of several important voices in the arena of team-building and motivating others, and hope to bring them together in the following section.

One of the most compelling reads in this area is *The Ideal Team Player: How to Recognize and Cultivate the Three Essential Virtues* by Patrick Lencioni (2016). Through the author's unique approach, I learned very quickly how to identify which characteristics most impact a team's configuration, and the importance of that configuration to the success of a manager or leader. Knowing those characteristics and identifying which team members display them clearly in the interview stage of team building is highly relevant and one that has not been emphasized sufficiently in the literature. Lencioni (2016) identifies humility, hunger, and smartness as the three major components of a good professional colleague. The author describes the importance and relevant underlying characteristics of these attributes.

He describes humble professionals as those who work for the greater good and satisfaction of professional goals established by an organization. Hungry professionals have the desire and are eager to participate, learn, and progress. Smart professionals are those who can understand the human dynamics of the team they work with. Good leaders, in my opinion, can work on these characteristics within themselves as well as foster them in others. Leaders must view each employee as having a combination of characteristics. The challenge is to understand and use these attributes for the good of team building and to promote progress.

The first place to begin team building is the organizational structure. Very few leaders walk into an organization and have the liberty of hiring and starting their own team from the ground up. Much more common is a novice leader who is hired to carry on an established department's goals, who must therefore learn on the job. There can be other more promising scenarios; for example, when a wise and experienced leader comes into a unit to lead it to a new objective or expand operations. This scenario has the advantage of pre-existing business savvy and "people smarts," or acumen. However, even this scenario has risks in that change takes time and simultaneously maintaining and growing operations is not for the faint of heart. Putting ego aside and taking a hard look at human resources as capital takes a great deal of personal investment and maturity. Many individuals with a more clinical background, for example, those with a career in identifying communication disabilities, simply do not have these more nebulous business aptitudes in their tool kit. In addition, identifying underlying dynamics can be a time-consuming task in that some of the subtler characteristics of individuals' work personalities may not reveal themselves until significant time has passed, and a project may fall short because of this.

What is the solution to this conundrum? "Taking a new broom and sweeping clean" is an old expression, but that is much easier said than done. Frequently, managers must seek opportunities to identify interpersonal relationship issues, to demonstrate exemplary behavior, and also initiate and capitalize on teachable moments. In many cases, this can be extremely hard to do in a fast-paced, results-oriented work environment. Also, seasoned employees may have been at the job longer than the new leader and may be suspicious and resistant to training that changes their pre-established work behaviors. The result, then, is a silo approach to program operations with limited inter-action beyond sharing procedural updates about what must get done, and not about the "hows" of team cohesion and growth.

The result of a stale approach such as this is that programs keep doing the same things in the same way. Individuals who do not achieve the satisfaction they aspire to may become com-plainers, become disgruntled, and eventually leave for another opportunity. Management expertise in effective team building could provide insight and address underlying issues before these outcomes result. In this case, the gathering of a team, pre-exist-ing or new, falls on the leader. The leader must have the cour-age to face the interpersonal dynamics of the department from the standpoint of both the individual members and the impact on the team as a whole. It takes a good deal of smarts to know what to say, how to say it, and when to say it; but there comes a time when a leader has to face this challenge, especially if a new endeavor is to be undertaken. Buy-in from team members is very challenging and engagement may be fleeting. However, the alternative is that team members stay and the fledgling manager seeks another job!

So why isn't the new broom approach taken more frequently, and why do managers prefer sometimes to do the work of the subordinates themselves instead of re-establishing the game rules?

The answer to this is obviously complicated. Managers work to establish themselves by aligning relationships within a team. They play to people's strengths. They frequently lead by example, and many are career-experienced individuals who can simply do the work of the team members rather than stimulating each member to contribute more. There are also hidden exog-enous factors in the pre-existing culture of a given workplace. For example, some environments outwardly value civility but do not seem to employ or reward it, which leads to less engage-ment in civil behaviors overall. Differing managerial styles across units (with some inherently less forward-thinking than others), leading to potentially damaging collateral communication that contaminates the goals of a fledgling department. People also tend to simply conform, rather than try to go against the tide. Leaders can become overwhelmed by lack of infrastructure or manpower, which can thwart implementation of new procedures. Navigating preexisting conditions while endeavoring new and meaningful projects is never an easy thing and takes an especially hardy manager.

In the current economy where all workers do more with less, it is understandable that leaders can become overwhelmed, and instead of sweeping changes, may make small in-roads for the next manager to build upon. Therefore, the idea of having many sources of personal and professional inspiration is especially meaningful in today's age. The very fact that now there may be up to five generations overlapping in one workplace setting requires unique strength to manage and maturity in team building. Wise managers seek to develop strength and maturity from many sources. As an example of current trends, speech pathologists can now gain exposure to more in-services and training on previously unstudied concepts such as emotional intelligence so they can monitor and focus work efforts externally and not feel depleted by directorial demands. For example, ASHA's convention in November 2017 in Los Angeles, California showcased a lecture given by Mary R. Reilly. Mary is the Director of Speech-Language Pathology Services at New York University Langone Medical Center in New York City, one of the largest and most prestigious departments in the world. She presented material highly relevant to all new and existing leaders and there is no substitute for learning in person. I support and encourage all readers to seek training in an in-person venue.

Another deeply important resource in our discipline is ASHA's Special Interest Group 11, focusing on issues related to Administration and Supervision. Other managers' resources and expertise apply well beyond student certification issues; their insights are a tremendous asset to directors of clinical education who may report to a senior centralized administrator, program director, or program chair. A big advantage is that Special Interest Group 11 is geared toward the profession, whereas other managerial forums may not be. An additional professional venue offering tremendous leadership training support is CAPCSD (Council on Programs in Communication Sciences and Disorders). These professional societies offer directors ready-made colleagues, educational presentations, and leadership training opportunities from individuals from all over the country who face similar issues.

Similarly, http://www.speechpathology.com provides seminars on topics of growing interest in supervision and administration, including the establishment of global best practices in the field. Grooming industry leaders is especially challenging given the globalization of the profession. The fact that many SLPs are interested in working abroad, and similarly, individuals come to the U.S. to establish careers and undergo training, demonstrates this global development. Continuing education opportunities continue to develop to meet the global demand for training in leadership skills.

A very substantial network of support for SLP directors seeking input is from seasoned training consortia. One such group that has been immeasurably supportive in my own career growth has been the Reality Based Leadership Group, headed by *New York Times* bestselling author, national keynote speaker, and consultant, Cy Wakeman. This group provides an immense range of information on recognizing leadership challenges and formulating strategies to confront them. Ms. Wakeman's group offers various platforms for learning through diverse scenarios that creatively address contemporary issues. Much of the basic information can be accessed freely via online videos (http://www.realitybasedleadership.com). For example, in one scenario, the goal is to identify overly dramatic staff members, who may be brilliant academically, but who force the department to deal with grandstanding and other issues that call for too much emotional handholding in the office, costing the department time and money. These individuals may not recognize that their behavior is disruptive. They may be very clever at diverting required work because they are excellent at analyzing and critiquing in a way that derails the tasks at hand. Overly dramatic professionals choose not to acknowledge that some of the challenges in any workplace involve getting things done despite outside circumstances. Wakeman talks about these challenges in a realistic way, and one in which I also believe, which is that some behaviors are more deeply rooted than a workplace can absorb and manage. This scenario calls for delicate and peaceful recognition that workplace and worker may no longer be a best fit. Recognizing this could require input from a professional human resource manager to find the best way to work toward expectations and consequences.

To focus on personal and interpersonal growth, leaders and managers can take classes from the Dale Carnegie training program. Many people from all walks of life have benefited from the written works, interactive workshops and personal coaching that the Carnegie program provides. The individual trainers are polished in approaches to managing expectations in the workplace, which may be half the battle in some organizations. The Carnegie program further affirms the importance of being open and flexible, engaging in life-long introspection, and identifying growth opportunities in oneself and one's team as integral to a vital and sustained workplace. Managers and leaders have typically worked very hard to achieve their status and their work merit is judged by skills sets they may not necessarily have formally studied. Grooming and sustaining areas of personal growth makes one's career a vital and evolving pathway as opposed to a dead end.

The ability to view a complex system from within and afar is necessary in order for leaders to form vision. Some organizations are able to hire consultants or have retreats, but rather than these occasional aids, it is the everyday tools and techniques that help managers remain in their role and experience the satisfaction of achievement. As previously stated, skills such as program evaluation and effective review techniques are independent abilities that are typically not studied in graduate school and beyond. The essential call to action for SLP directors are to avail themselves of, and integrate into, the world of business acumen so that departments are administered by professionals in the field and not people who are uneducated in the end product of speech services delivery. We as a profession, if we want to ensure SLPs are prescribing our program strategies, have to be smart and specific about the strategic plans we present, so that we are fully confident in the business and administrative skills required for the formulation of such strategies. When a lack of training or professional knowledge is identified, using allied professionals and understanding current lifestyle philosophies are helpful to the engaged manager. Undoubtedly, the work and skills I've described call for extra effort and thought outside of the workplace, which is a growing challenge as we face downturns in the medical and educational economies, both in the United States and worldwide. Self-help practices such as yoga and meditation focus on introspection, which leads to the identification of self-strengths and weaknesses. Thinkers such as Marianne Williamson, whose philosophies focus on peacebuilding and acceptance, help nourish leaders as they integrate or build their programs for the coming years. The reputation of a program depends on its leader putting a face to it, and on having the vision and support necessary to carry out its goals.

It is critical that developing leaders appreciate the depth and scope of their responsibilities, both assigned and inherent in the leadership role. The designation of *leader* is a call to develop ones personal best using a multitude of available resources and strategies and through creative appreciation of personal reflection and growth. It is clear that recruitment and retention of high-level management personnel is a delicate undertaking in human services, and involves individuals, teams, the workplace, and societal influences to create an effective environment in which all components can flourish. The combination of professional and personal resources help individuals both start, as well as mature, in a leadership trajectory.

Reflection

Where does leadership emerge from? What can supportive mentorship and effective teams contribute?

References

Carozza, L. (2010). *Science of successful supervision and mentorship.* San Diego, CA: Plural.

Feldman, H. (2018). Identifying, building, and sustaining your leadership team. *Journal of Professional Nursing, 34,* 87–91. https://doi .org/10.1016/j.profnurs.2017.11.002

Groupthink. (2018). In *Merriam-Webster online dictionary.* Retrieved from https://www.merriam-webster.com/dictionary/groupthink

Hougaard, R., Carter, J., & Afton, M. (2018, January 12). Self-awareness can help leaders more than an MBA can. *Harvard Business Review.*

Retrieved from https://hbr.org/2018/01/self-awareness-can-help-leaders-more-than-an-mba-can

Lencioni, P. (2016). *The ideal team player: How to recognize and cultivate the three essential virtues.* Hoboken, NJ: Wiley.

Pilling, S., & Slattery, J. (2004). Management competencies: Intrinsic or acquired? What competencies are required to move into speech-pathology management and beyond? *Australian Health Review, 27*(1), 84–92. https://doi.org/10.1071/AH042710084

Additional Resource

Speech-Pathology. (n.d.). Continuing education. Retrieved from https://www.speechpathology.com/

5

Internal and External Problem-Solving

Linda S. Carozza

A problem is only a problem if you refuse to look for a solution. If you don't take action to fix it then it will remain a problem.

—Catherine Pulsifer

Learning Objective

- Readers will learn about the structure of problem-solving: asking the right questions, assessing the contributing and maintaining factors, and designing strategies for short-term and long-term intervention.

Introduction

In the previous chapters, we discussed some of the basics of leadership and some of the potential pitfalls, unexpected factors and influences brought about by a setting's various cultural components, and legislative or managerial aspects of leadership in particular landscapes. In addition, we outlined some of the personal and professional characteristics that may impact leadership opportunities and growth.

In this chapter, the goal is to discuss various-aspects of leadership that can underlie or affect the growth of emergent leaders. The primary framework is a description of four styles of leaders, and how the differences between styles in problem-solving approaches affects team building. The view of Johnson Vickberg and Christfort (2018) is highly relevant to leadership language that can guide the understanding and development of teams.

A common challenge for organizations is insightful and directive leadership, particularly as it applies to effective problem-solving. New hires may be brought in to implement the agendas of pre-existing or even newly developed strategic plans, only to be replaced a few years later by others with more vision. Why should a perfectly good group of professionals not be able to keep its eye on an agenda and bring it to fruition? What might underlie changeovers in management that stall goal achievement and cost organizations meaningful growth? These challenges affect everyone from the boardroom to the "boots on the ground" staff, who may all feel the impact of stalled projects and derailed initiatives (that return packaged as new initiatives) when fresh leadership repeatedly takes the reins. All too often this leads to organizations become stale and to lack the vibrancy and growth that may have attracted new managers in the first place.

Discussion

Leadership education frequently includes an introduction to industry psychology after managers are already in place, which can lead to managerial failure to thrive or meet preset goals. Training after a manager is already in place ignores the need for business personalities to be understood before managers set foot in the conference room.

Johnson Vickberg and Christfort (2018) initially developed an extensive inventory of 1000 professionals in each of three independent samples. Using various statistical models in their final sample of more than 190,000 individuals allowed them to propose work-style personality standards and discuss overarching factors that affect those standards, such as the influence of stress. This information can help managers who strive to be the best leaders of corporations and industry. The authors continue their work in interactive sessions with companies who field test and refine the models to face work challenges and growth more effectively and efficiently.

Although each leader represents a mix of work personalities, there is a tendency for each to be more oriented toward one of four composite work personalities developed by Johnson Vickberg and Christfort (2018): pioneers, guardians, drivers, and integrators. Personality characteristics describe what motivates or challenges workers and how their thinking patterns and approach to problem-solving differ across individuals. Armed with this knowledge, groups can better understand how to assign and accomplish tasks, and how to reach consensus with a more meaningful perspective.

A Summary of Each Style

- Pioneers are innovative in their thinking and are drawn to the possibilities in a situation. They value risks for the benefits they may provide. They have energy and imagination.
- Guardians value stability and order in a pragmatic sense. They work with data and measurements, and look for detail and to learn from the past.
- Drivers value change and momentum. They are results- and goal-driven. They may work with logic and data, and view issues head-on.
- Integrators value team building and making connections. They value relationships in groups and are diplomatic and consensus minded.

When a group understands and embraces their work strengths, they can better tackle problems rather than harbor disagreement with each other. Leaders should match tasks that need to be accomplished with the people who are best able to accomplish them. This compass of shared purpose or "rowing in the same direction" is an essential place for all leaders to begin from, although, it is sometimes hard to navigate to that point due to preexisting challenges.

The benefit of understanding one's teams cannot be overstated. In order to stimulate a team to utilize the strengths of its different personality styles, leaders must pull opposites closer and garner input from all, including those with nondominant personalities. In the same vein, introverted thinkers who have a lot to contribute but do not speak out must be encouraged and supported, or their many valuable insights can be lost when dominant personalities take over a meeting. Trust and respect for individual differences and strengths are hallmarks of a well-developed team and successful leaders.

Another strategy that can assist in leadership building is to have the various personality types work on smaller projects at first to help engender partnerships. Leaders also must know how to pull their own opposites close to them; therefore, self-analysis of how one interacts in different settings and with different levels is key.

Literature described by the *Harvard Business Review* reports when highest-level administrators are surveyed, most top leaders are pioneers or drivers. These pioneers and drivers are the officers of corporations, or so-called C-suite executives (i.e., CEO, COO, CFO, etc.). The next highest-level leaders are guardians, followed by integrators. A danger of this hierarchy, however, is that top-down thinking may cascade to lower-level managers, who then do not contribute as effectively as they might have in a less hierarchical model. A group may succumb to a groupthink mentality and not benefit from the broader perspective and contributions of individuals.

Teams can find themselves dominated by one or another style, and good leaders seek to balance their teams, perhaps by calling in a team building expert, or having a retreat or other out-of-the-office activity with equal numbers of personality types represented and comfortably for the individual and collective benefit of all. A common pitfall, however, is that individuals with dominant personalities may not be amenable to change or cooperation, feeling that they know what is needed and how to accomplish specific goals. A challenge of new leaders, then, is how to draw out the best in your team, how to get everyone's buy-in and reduce pushback from the more dominant types.

This is particularly challenging for new managers or leaders of a well-established group, that has worked together for a long time, regardless of whether they were interpersonally successful or productive. Also, organizational pressures may be such that many projects are due at once and quality is sacrificed for the quantity of products for which a unit is responsible. Some more obvious factors affecting team cohesiveness are age, gender, and culture, but less perceptible aspects can affect the organizational environment as well. For example, goals that require procedures with long learning curves can also affect how a team works together. To avoid turnover and bouncing from position to position, leaders are best armed with knowledge about individual work personalities and respect for the value of communication, both with individuals and within groups.

A challenge in most office scenarios is how to achieve this delicate balance, and then to grow and retain respect of your colleagues and peers. To avoid marginalization of important team contributions, leaders should give thoughtful, introverted members time to consider the details of a project and give them the necessary tools to prepare for the discussion and solution phase. For example, allow less vocal members to contribute ideas in writing, as opposed to taking the floor at a meeting. An option for members who think on their feet and are fast to respond, the so-called pioneers, is to make advanced reading and preparation an option rather than a requirement, which goes along with their desire for spontaneity.

In order for all team members to benefit from the collective thinking styles, some leaders use large collaborative flip charts or chalkboards to generate and encourage as many ideas as possible in an open forum style. This allows expansive thinkers in the group an opportunity to provide big picture ideas and also encourages detail-oriented thinkers on the team to contribute equally in a more informal environment than a typical meeting room setting. Another customization that can be helpful is disseminating information for a particular aspect of the meeting so that expectations can be shared and managed more clearly. It also helps if some of the background work for a discussion can be done by the leader or staff members before a meeting to reduce anxieties and allow time for perspectives to develop during meetings. A good leader knows when to deliver information, how much information to deliver and what format deliver it in. Suffice it to say that leaders gain these pearls of wisdom from many perspectives over multiple work settings, and can be communicated, but not truly integrated, except via hands-on training and going through example exercises or simulations. Increased mentorships or managerial internships are useful in non-corporate industries to mirror the training of business models hands-on training and examples.

Fast-paced team members will want discussions to maintain a brisk pace with clear links to solutions, as opposed to focusing on building consensus. It is important to try to build and strengthen relationships between individuals who value different work styles although it takes an additional skill set to learn what motivates each person and group to buy in. In general, strategies work best when all opinions are heard before moving forward. If your goal is efficient opinion sharing based on learned information, rather than conducting education at a meeting, it's helpful for group members to educate themselves before meetings about the topics to be discussed. In addition, leaders playing devil's advocate to propose alternative viewpoints evoke new thinking in members when they see the challenges a particular decision creates. This can jump-start not only new thinking and conversation, but can also help reduce reactions that take place after the meeting that could sabotage moving ahead with decisions.

There is an old saying that a chain is only as strong as its weakest link. Thus, a wise leader makes sure that even the most quiet team members are heard. Because some of the group may be younger or intimidated by the group for whatever reason, it is important to seek out and embrace divergent opinions, particularly from members who appear risk-averse. Johnson Vickberg and Christfort (2018) cautioned leaders to learn about the effects of stress on a team. Each personality type on your team will be affected by stress in a different manner. These effects may come in the form of face-to-face discussions, conflicts in meetings, or a sense of institutional urgency about certain projects. In today's workplace, regardless if it is in the private or public sector, the pace of work is very fast and can be highly competitive and challenging for almost any personality type at one time or another. An interesting juxtaposition arises here: do managers take time to work with highly conscientious workers who are susceptible to stress? Research suggests that they should, as some of the most engaged and intuitive workers are those who see the details of situations but do not speak up (Cain, 2012). In particular, this applies to workers with social or performance anxiety, the stress of which may leave them silent when solicited for ideas or opinions. Those with anxiety about the scope of a project may be able to work on individual portions–with depth and tenacity, and drawing them in while honoring the differences and similarities in your team will pay off. Slowing the pace of discussions, itemizing meeting agendas, and in general, finding ways to support different workstyles are all ways to support the professionals you lead or manage. According to Susan Cain's popular TED Talk (2018), it is time to stop defaulting to group work and consider that some tasks are better done in solitude and reported back to the larger group! It is important, too, not to catch more diffident team members off-guard, but rather, give them time and space to reflect in advance and then voice their opinions. This adjustment makes for more comfortable meetings. Just as with children we instruct as educators, teams work best when they are psychologically secure. A sense of security helps generate ideas and allows them to blossom. With attention to the inherent strengths of the different thinking styles of your group members, you can make the most of your time by benefiting from their diversity and culling it to get a product that reflects the best of each type. You can get the big picture and also work out the details! The umbrella of an expansive thinker allows resource-oriented staff on your team to feel comfortable and that their jobs are meaningful. It is up to us the leaders to learn leadership skills, enhance our own strategies, and model for others the best of the best for the goals of any entity to be met and flourish.

Effective Problem-Solving Techniques

There are specific techniques for effective problem-solving, regardless of differences in working style. These proven techniques facilitate achieving goals by minimizing the occurrence of disruptive internal problems. Many posit that problem-solving ability, in fact, may be the most important defining characteristic of great leaders (Ancona & Gregersen, 2018; Llopis, 2013). At Forbes, Glenn Llopis (2013) listed the techniques below as the four most effective ways that leaders solve problems. According to Llopis, they help leaders view problems as opportunities, rather than hindrances, and allow leaders to employ *circular vision*, or broadened observation: the ability to see problems from all sides.

- Communicate transparently: The ability of a leader to engender communication from all team members has been previously discussed in this chapter. It is ironic, especially for leaders within a communications sciences field, that communication is often viewed as so fundamental that its importance is overlooked. Leaders may have to use nuanced intuition to achieve transparent communication, especially because people may not always be comfortable sharing their true thoughts or feelings.
- Break down silos: The silo mentality, as defined by BusinessDictionary.com (2019) is "a mind-set present in some companies when certain departments or sectors do not wish to share information with others in the same company." This definition can easily be applied to many other sectors, all the way down to individuals within the same organization. Workplace silos are often constructed by self-promoting employees, and may suggest hidden agendas. Silos can hinder open communication and team building.
- Remain open-minded: Combining the first two techniques helps encourage open-mindedness. Actively listening to another's concerns and exposure to differing viewpoints, particularly from those whom you respect in a work environment, is key to developing open-mindedness. Open-minded individuals are more likely to see past personal differences and tackle problems head-on to the benefit of the organization and all involved.
- Embrace a solid foundational strategy: This refers back to the idea that without vision, an organization may find itself doing the same (incorrect) things the same (ineffective) way. That is, substituting, not evolving. A founda-

tional strategy allows leaders to see the overall map of a problem, thus viewing a problem from all sides, and to plot specific actions accordingly.

The Importance of Problem-Solving in a Leadership Position

Current literature supports the idea that problem-solving ability is perhaps the most important quality integral to an effective leader (Ancona & Gregerson, 2018). Vivienne Ming, a technology leader, MIT alumnus, and an individual lauded in her field for her ability to think openly and assemble talent, says "the only reason I do it [being a problem-led leader] is because it is an amazingly effective way to have an impact on the world" (Ancona & Gregerson, 2018). For those in speech-language pathology, impacting the world for better seems an inherent goal, and one worthy of cultivation. Current research also suggests problem-led leadership is a general trend worldwide, and will continue to be important for future leadership development.

Conclusion

It is beyond the scope of this book to describe how to accomplish personal reflection and growth. However, recruitment and retention of high-level management personnel in human services is a delicate undertaking, and involves the individual, the team, the workplace, and societal influences to create an effective environment in which all components flourish.

Reflection

What are some ways that problem-solving skills can be developed and sharpened so leaders can construct proactive strategies to deal with organizational objectives?

References

Ancona, D., & Gregersen, H. (2018, April 16). *The power of leaders who focus on solving problems.* Retrieved from https://hbr.org/2018/04/the-power-of-leaders-who-focus-on-solving-problems

Cain, S. (2012, February). *The power of introverts* [Video file]. Retrieved from https://www.ted.com/talks/susan_cain_the_power_of_introverts

Johnson Vickberg, S. M., & Christfort, K. (2018, March–April). Pioneers, drivers, integrators and guardians. *Harvard Business Review,* 5056. Retrieved from https://hbr.org/2017/03/the-new-science-of-team-chemistry#pioneers-drivers-integrators-and-guardians

Llopis, G. (2013, November 4). The 4 most effective ways leaders solve problems. *Forbes.* Retrieved from https://www.forbes.com/sites/glennllopis/2013/11/04/the-4-most-effective-ways-leaders-solve-problems/#36f861aa4f97

Silo mentality. (2019). In *Business Dictionary.com.* Retrieved from http://www.businessdictionary.com/definition/silo-mentality.html

Additional Resources

Lencioni, P. (2016). *The ideal team player: How to recognize and cultivate the three essential virtues.* Hoboken, NJ: Wiley.

Speech-Pathology: Continuing Education. (n.d.). Retrieved from https://www.speechpathology.com/

6

Testing Leadership

Linda S. Carozza

> *We can deny everything, except the*
> *possibility that we can be better.*
>
> —Dalai Lama

Learning Objective

- To provide real-life case scenarios so that readers can apply their insights as emergent and developing leaders. Discussions surrounding appropriate combinations of actions for each scenario may develop, and such discussions are encouraged.

Scenario 1

Your employee is treating an 8-year-old boy for specific language impairment at a private clinic for speech-language pathology and audiology in a rural community. The boy and his family recently relocated from out of town. The parent is a second grade school teacher and is the sole legal guardian of the child. The child currently receives individual speech-language therapy services at the clinic. Therapy goals include resolution of his use of double negatives and zero copula during speech. The child's mother communicates in an English dialect that is different from that of the therapist. She asks the therapist to discontinue the above therapy goals because she feels that her child's language differences are being misinterpreted as a language disorder. The therapist consults with the parent and tells her that her child needs this therapy, and that she has no right to refuse consent. The therapist continues to administer therapy with the goal of treating his dialect, despite ongoing parental protest. The parent remains frustrated but eventually concedes, because this is the only pediatric clinic available in the immediate area. The parent has written an official complaint to you, the clinic administrator, in hopes of resolving the situation.

As a Leader in This Speech-Language Pathology Clinic, What Should You Do?

1. Do not support the parent. Convey to her the importance of her child complying with treatment and achieving the goals outlined by the therapist. Continuing therapy without any changes to the plan of care is in the best interest of the child. Explain to the parent that without following these clinical recommendations, her child may not be able to achieve the best functional outcome.

2. Consult with the therapist and parent individually. Convey to the therapist the importance of cultural sensitivity in developing treatment goals. Encourage her to reassess her clinical judgment, and to consider the possibility that some of the child's language deficits are in fact, a part of his normal dialect. Ask her to modify her treatment goals accordingly, in collaboration with the child and parent. Facilitate a new consultation between the therapist and parent. If the therapist refuses, take disciplinary action for her refusal to respect the patient's bill of rights, and immediately assign a new therapist to the patient.

3. Discontinue speech-language therapy services for the child until a new therapist can be assigned. Place the

therapist on administrative leave and inform the parent that her child has been placed on a waiting list until further notice.

Evaluating the Responses

1. This is not the correct response. The parent should receive support from the clinical staff for sharing her comments and concerns. Although it is important for health care providers to encourage their patients and families to continue treatment whenever it is clinically recommended, it is equally important to understand that patients (or the parents of child patients) have the legal right to refuse treatment for non-life-threatening conditions. Specific language impairment (SLI) falls under the category of a non-life-threatening illness. Seeking to impose any treatment, or even specific aspects of treatment, without the informed consent of the patient or his parent violates the patient's bill of rights. In this case, there is no reason to believe that the parent is incompetent, and her refusal to provide consent for treatment cannot legally be contested by the therapist.

2. This is the correct response. The therapist should employ cultural sensitivity in developing her treatment goals for her patient. In addition, the SLP must be aware of language differences in her clinical populations. She may conduct a new evaluation, possibly using diagnostic tests and diagnostic materials that are more sensitive to dialectical features. The therapist should consult with the parent in a clinician-patient relationship model that accommodates patient autonomy, patient values, and ongoing information disclosure with regard to treatment. Understanding the patient's cultural and language identity is important in deciding the course of treatment. In addition, the therapist may receive disciplinary action for her lack of knowledge regarding informed parental consent. She may be advised to review the patient's bill of rights in order to avoid any future violations and litigation from other patients.

3. This is not the correct response. Although the therapist may not have employed good communication with the parent, and appeared to lack cultural sensitivity in her clinical evaluation of the patient, discontinuing therapy without some attempt at mediation will be a disservice to the child, especially because there are limited pediatric services available in this community. Discontinuation of services may make it difficult for the parent and child to seek appropriate treatment. The clinic should continue therapy services for the child without interruption, but in a way that respects the parent's decisions during treatment.

Scenario 2

You are the executive director of a nonprofit multidisciplinary clinic in the inner city. This is a community-based clinic that accepts both insured patients, and uninsured patients with sliding fee scales. As such, your clinic has an extensive caseload and is grossly understaffed. Some of your patients have been on a waiting list for several months. Your speech-language pathologists are particularly burdened with an extremely high caseload and extensive backlog. You are unable to hire additional workers due to a limited budget for new hires. Some of your current patients have filed complaints with the front desk about extensive waiting times in the clinic. If you do not act soon, many of your current and prospective patients will look for an alternative clinic, leading to a loss in revenue. You may have to make changes to your current staff.

As the Executive Director of This Community-Based Clinic, What Should You Do?

1. Do not change your staff. Your employees have been working in this clinic for many years. They are well-known by the patients and the local community. Any downsizing will affect the company culture and under-

mine the rapport established by your clinicians with their patients.

2. Contract your clinicians and hire assistants. By offering contract positions to your clinicians, you may be able to reduce costs relating to workers benefits and salaries. Propose fair contract offers to clinicians who have been working for a shorter period of time or who have other commitments outside of work. If multiple clinicians are contracted, as opposed to salaried, use the surplus in your budget to hire part-time speech-language pathology assistants at an hourly rate.

3. Decreasing the time period for each therapy session by 20% and schedule additional patients into the weekly schedule. Clinicians will be expected to accommodate more patients in their daily schedule in the hopes that waiting time for patients in the clinic will be substantially reduced.

Evaluating the Responses

1. This is not the correct response. Although maintaining the same staff is helpful in building long-term clinician-patient relationships, staff cohesion, and company morale, many of the patients will inadvertently suffer because of extended waiting times in the clinic and long waiting lists for appointments. Timely therapy is especially important for patients who have an acquired illness (e.g., poststroke aphasia). Without an early response, some patients may not fully recover or be able to maximize their functional outcome due to lost time.

2. This is the correct response. Contractual and per-diem employment is a developing trend in all industries, including the medical one (Noguchi, 2018). Contracting employees helps to control costs and allows more flexibility with work schedules and staff placement, compared to traditional salaried workers. It also helps employers by adding more employees to handle the workload, if schedules are organized appropriately. Decreasing the number of salaried workers with benefits,

while increasing the number of part-time, contracted clinicians and paraprofessionals, will help to efficiently manage the caseload, decrease waiting times, and reduce costs. It will also help to increase revenue over time. Consider hiring a part-time grants administrator to organize development and fundraising activities on behalf of the clinic, in order to further increase the budget for future hires or even add additional days or hours of operation to the clinic schedule.

3. This is not the correct response. Although many clinics and hospitals are moving toward a model of shorter and fewer therapy sessions (Mullen & Schooling, 2010), this has profound implications for treatment efficacy. This is an ongoing debate in speech-language pathology. Research shows that treatment efficacy may depend on the frequency and intensity of treatment. However, treatment schedules should always be adjusted to the population (i.e., child, adult, or senior) or the type of communicative disorder treated, so in effect, there is no specific blueprint for how a treatment schedule should look (Nippold, 2012). Nevertheless, in an ideal world, clinicians should always have the option of increasing therapy time or therapy visits whenever warranted.

Scenario 3

You are a speech-language pathology Department Chair at a large hospital with a diverse staff in a multicultural community known for high levels of immigration. Your newly hired licensed speech therapist, Mr. X, told his direct supervisor that he would need to observe prayers during a workday prior to seeing one of his patients next week. The day is not a major holiday in his religion, nor is it noted on any workplace calendar. He asks for this accommodation and requests permission to reschedule his first patient at a later time. The supervisor approves his request and tells him not to worry; she will let everyone know.

The following week, Mr. X arrives to work on time, and proceeds to engage in religious prayer on the day for which he requested accommodation. His patient arrives earlier than expected and demands to see him right then due to other pending medical appointments. He complains to the receptionist about Mr. X. The receptionist apologizes, and realizes that she had forgotten to reschedule the patient at a later time. Coincidentally, Mr. X's supervisor called in sick and an alternate supervisor arrives, finding Mr. X in his office in prayer. She opens and slams his door and yells an expletive in the hallway, making an inflammatory remark against his religious identity. No one heard what she said but Mr. X. As Mr. X walks out to find out what she wanted, she turns arounds and sternly tells him that he should be seeing his patient. She subsequently files a complaint against Mr. X with human resources and demands that he take a leave of absence. You receive a copy of the complaint from this supervisor in your inbox.

As the Departmental Chair of This City Hospital, What Should You Do?

1. Discipline Mr. X. Disciplinary action against your employee should be taken with an oral and written warning provided to Mr. X in an in-office meeting. Mr. X should also be advised not to engage in religious activity in his office during working hours. Explain the following to him: His actions were unethical in that he neglected his required clinical responsibilities to follow private religious observances. In addition, he participated in a religious practice that was not even a part of a major religious holiday. More importantly, his patient was seen later than the patient expected and had no choice but to cancel his other medical appointments. This caused a major inconvenience for his patient, raising ethical questions regarding Mr. X's clinical competency. He also caused financial hardship to the hospital, due to a sudden shift in the daily schedule and potential loss of revenue from his disgruntled patient.
2. Discipline the supervisors. The first supervisor was responsible for orientating Mr. X to workplace policies and procedures regarding religious observances.

Do not discipline the receptionist, she was not at fault because Mr. X's planned religious observance was not directly communicated to her. Discipline the second supervisor for her unprofessional behavior, which can be considered as discriminatory in nature. The fact that Mr. X was practicing religious prayer that was not required by his religion is irrelevant. Mr. X is free to practice his religion whenever he wishes, so long as he asks for a reasonable accommodation. In this case, he did ask for an accommodation.

Evaluating the Responses

1. This is not the correct response. According to federal and state law, employers may not harass employees based on religious beliefs or practices. The supervisor was wrong to slam Mr. X's office door and verbally harass him, whatever the reason. Her actions can be described as workplace harassment and discrimination. In addition, employers must make reasonable accommodations for affirmed religious beliefs. Rescheduling a patient is not outside the norm of typical operations in a hospital clinic, especially with advanced notice. Mr. X had asked to reschedule this patient a week prior, and it likely would not have created hardship for the patient had his supervisor communicated this to all appropriate staff. The employer is at fault in this situation and is liable for workplace discrimination and violation of religious rights in the workplace, due to its failure to reasonably accommodate Mr. X's religious observances, which was in fact, already granted by one of his supervisors.

2. This is the correct response. Mr. X changing his work schedule in order to pray on a specific day and time is an example of an accommodation for religious practice. Although employers are not required to provide such accommodations, employers are expected to respect such observances if the request is granted, as it was

in this case. In addition, state law requires employers to allow their employees to observe holy days, unless a religious observance would cause the employer an undue hardship, such as a significant financial loss. The employer suffered no such loss as a result of Mr. X's actions in this situation. Whatever loss was incurred was a direct result of a communication breakdown between supervisory and administrative staff. Mr. X took the appropriate course of action by requesting an accommodation in advance, specifically, a schedule change, and by indicating that he would need time on a specific day and at a specific time for religious observance. Employers are required to at least attempt to accommodate various religious practices, including prayer on a workday. Mr. X is not at fault for his religious observance in the workplace, although his patient should receive an apology and be rescheduled for a new appointment as soon as possible. His supervisor should receive training in multicultural competency with a focus on religious diversity, and be monitored for any behaviors that appear to qualify as workplace discrimination. If her misbehavior continues, she should be terminated due to her violation of workers' rights.

The employer could be held liable for not taking appropriate action in this case.

Scenario 4

You are the owner of a multidisciplinary medical clinic in City X that includes pediatricians, SLPs, and developmental psychologists. Your clinic is known for specializing in autism treatment. One of your speech therapists is a homosexual male who is well-known for his political activism in the community and respected for his professionalism and clinical expertise in autism spectrum disorder. He often wears a subtle rainbow-colored wristband to work to express his pride in supporting the gay community. The wristband is typically covered by his long sleeve dress shirt, but might be exposed on occasion. After being assigned a 9-year-old boy with autism, the clinician introduced himself to the parents and proceeded with conducting therapy. The boy's father appeared distressed and uncomfortable with the therapist. After the therapy session ended, the therapist walked the boy back into the waiting room, leaned over and gently touching him on the shoulder, telling the child, "You did an awesome job today! Remember to do your homework. Hope to see you again tomorrow, okay?" The father saw the interaction. He quickly got off his chair and yelled "Hey! Stop touching my son! I knew you were a [expletive]!" The clinician looked bewildered. The boy felt stunned. The mother began crying and the father proceeded to file a complaint with the clinic for sexual harassment.

As the Owner and Manager of This Private Clinic, What Should You Do?

1. Carefully review and file the complaint. Compile all notes from the complainant and the accused. Then report the incident to your human resources director for a prompt investigation. Temporarily put the child's case on hold. Place the clinician on paid leave.
2. Terminate the clinician. Apologize to the patient's family for this incident. Immediately transfer the child to another clinician.
3. Remove the patient and his family from the clinic. Apologize to the clinician and ban the patient from receiving any services at your clinic due to his father's behavior.

Evaluating the Responses

1. This is the correct response. Managers are legally responsible for handling all cases of sexual harassment no matter how minor or questionable they may seem. Placing the clinician on paid leave and the child's case on a temporary hold is a safe way to proceed with the investigation while preventing any other altercations between the clinician and the patient's family.

After concluding the investigation and establishing the facts of this case, the clinic should sincerely apologize to the clinician. Human resources may close the case. The clinician should be allowed to practice and continue his caseload. Explain to him that the clinic recognizes that the father was wrong in treating him unfairly, and in falsely accusing him of sexual harassment. The investigation concluded that the father's behavior was indicative of his discriminatory attitude toward homosexuals. Transfer the child to another clinician to avoid any further contact between the clinician and the child's family. You must advocate for treating the child despite his father's behavior. You may not have the grounds to remove the patient from the clinic based on his father's behavior in this case, as the father did not violently threaten the clinician or any other staff. If he continues to behave inappropriately, the father may have to be permanently barred from the clinic, at which time the mother, or any other legal guardian can accompany the child to the clinic. You may want to hold a staff meeting. Inform staff that this is a discrimination-free workplace, and that the clinic values the diversity of its team. In addition, inform staff that they may have to interact with patients and families who may discriminate against them according to race, religion, or sexual orientation. This is an unfortunate part of human interaction, but clinicians must put their patients first, and work in the best interest of their patients despite any hostility that the patients (or their families) harbor toward clinicians because of their backgrounds. However, emphasize that any behavior from visitors that appears to be threatening or violent will not be tolerated and will be grounds for removal from the clinic.

2. This is not the correct response. No disciplinary action should be taken until all facts are known. No investigation has been conducted and the clinic should not be biased toward the patient or the clinician. The manager should be neutral in handling these complaints. All evidence should be considered. Both parties and any witnesses to the incident should be interviewed. The

clinic will be at risk for a wrongful termination lawsuit if a manager fires the clinician.

3. This is not the correct response. Although the patient's father was clearly discriminating against the clinician, he was not in any way threatening the clinician with violence. The clinic does not have the legal right to screen patients and their families according to their social or political views. The clinic should only take legal action against the father if he continues to harass the clinician. The clinic should always consider the rights of the patient, and put his interests first. Although this incident created an uncomfortable workplace, it would be a great disservice to the child if he were to be transferred to another clinic. He may not have access to autism experts in other parts of the city. His treatment outcome may be poor without continuing treatment. The child must be the priority. The father may have to be consulted in order to help reduce the tension.

Reflection

Is leadership different in different contexts? What are some of the overarching themes of leadership? What are some aspects that must be case-specific for the best outcomes to emerge?

References

Mullen, R., & Schooling, T. (2010). The national outcomes measurement system for pediatric speech-language pathology. *Language, Speech and Hearing Services in schools, 41*(1), 44–60. https://doi.org/10.1044/0161-1461(2009/08-0051)

Nippold, M. A. (2012). Different service delivery methods for different communication disorders. *Language, Speech and Hearing Services in Schools, 43*(2),117. https://doi.org/10.1044/0161-1461(2012/ed-02)

Noguchi, Y. (2018). Freelanced: The rise of the contract worker. Retrieved from https://www.npr.org/2018/01/22/578825135/rise-of-the-contract-workers-work-is-different-now

Additional Resources

How Much Treatment Is Enough? (2015). Retrieved from https://www
.theinformedslp.com/qa_intensity.html

New York State Attorney General. (n.d.). *Religious rights in the workplace* [Brochure]. Retrieved from https://ag.ny.gov/sites/default/
files/religious_rights_in_the_workplace.pdf

7

Negotiation, Politics, and the Concept of Power

Linda S. Carozza
with acknowledgment to Katie LaForce

Patience is power. Patience is not an absence of action; rather it is 'timing.' It waits on the right time to act, for the right principles and in the right way.
—Fulton J. Sheen

Learning Objective

- To outline the concept of *power* in social interactions involving the workplace and to discuss related strategies to increase the awareness and skill set of new and emergent leaders.

Introduction

Power dynamics exist in every field. Effective leaders have to navigate the waters of power and politics with poise. Regardless of how cohesive a faculty or department may be, conflict—and therefore conflict management—is always a part of the package. Leaders in academia, medical settings, and other administrative positions encounter difficulties between employees and themselves, between employees and other employees, and even between themselves and their own supervisors. Leaders have to decide when and where to give way to the ideas of others or to draw a line. These situations call for ample negotiation skills. This section covers several strategies for negotiation that can aid in assessing and diffusing tense situations in the workplace.

Power in the Workplace

Power comes in many forms, and in both formal and informal varieties. Depending on the makeup of a work environment, each form is used in different proportions and with differing efficacy. Leaders, whether professors, administrators, or health care team leaders, need an apt understanding of the basis and use of each variety.

The Kinds of Organizational Power

Natter (2018) describes five kinds of power found in business models: coercive, legitimate, reward, referent, and expert power. Because the CSD field requires even its paraprofessionals to have a bachelor's degree, almost all employees or team members exude some form of expert power. Individual specialties and additional certifications stratify expert power.

Power as a Form of Capital

It is important when building a nurturing and productive environment to assess how power is perceived. Many people view power as a limited source. This line of thinking assumes that one can only gain power by taking it from someone else. This perspective can be very dangerous to the cohesiveness of a work team. Therefore, it is prudent for leaders to proactively create an environment that encourages free and open dialogue among team members. Open dialogue creates an atmosphere where power is considered to be a personal gain and not a spoil of war.

The Power of Feedback

Leaders sometimes avoid giving feedback, which is problematic for two reasons. First, positive feedback is encouraging to employees. Behavior analysis shows that positive reinforcement increases the likelihood that a targeted behavior will happen again (Skinner, 1938). It is imperative that leaders use this knowledge to their advantage. When leaders give employees social praise or other incentive, employees will continue that wanted behavior. Examples include rewarding employees for turning in paperwork on time or implementing new workplace protocols. Second, many workers want to do well at their chosen profession; however, improving job performance depends highly upon periodic review of achievement. It is difficult for an employee to fix a problem if he or she is unaware that it exists in the first place. By giving constructive feedback to team members, leaders capitalize on their worker's current productivity and give them opportunity for improvement and possible advancement.

The Power of "We"

When giving feedback to employees or students, the way that we frame conversations can greatly influence how feedback is received, and in turn, acted on. Framing a situation as a challenge for both you and your subordinates implies that you are helping employees find and implement solutions. Similarly, this route avoids an us versus them mentality, in favor of a more collaborative and professionally nurturing attitude.

The Power of Inclusion

In the United States, affirmative action with regard to business uses employment-related practices, such as recruitment, hiring, training, promotions, and termination to remedying the effects of past discrimination. Many employers achieve equity and diversity through means other than formal affirmative action measures. Still, certain federal government contractors must adhere to regulations enforced by the U.S. Department of Labor. An example of affirmative action is including efforts to increase the pool of qualified candidates from diverse groups in an organization's recruitment practices. Affirmative actions such as these can be characterized as de jure inclusion (required by law) or de facto inclusion (existing, but not required by law). In normal circumstances, de jure is a superfluous term, because organizations seek to function via all government statutes, particularly organizations that receive governmental financial aid.

The Power of Diversity

This leads to the notion of collective voices for strategizing and developing leadership plans in organizations that value multiple perspectives and points of view to engender the highest levels of efficiency and efficacy. Diverse faculty or employee bodies improves overall cultural competency in the workplace and improves workplace cohesion and overall well-being of clients and services that a program provides.

Conflict Management

Invariably, however, conflict arises in every organization. Before conflict resolution can begin, the situation surrounding the problem must be appropriately assessed. Duggan (n.d.) suggests using a root cause analysis technique for this purpose. Begin by identifying five possible causes, or roots, that led to conflict. The analysis can be put together based on input from the parties involved in the conflict, whether it is an interpersonal conflict or a conflict of party interests, or from more objective third parties. Be sure to follow the trail all the way to the end, as it would only be a short-term solution to treat the symptoms and not the roots.

Interpersonal Conflicts

When dealing specifically with conflict between people, it is important to ask questions to clarify the situation. By choosing to listen, leaders gain facts to apply to the resolution and avoid being perceived as accusatory or apathetic to others' perspectives. Garfinkle (2017) gives five tips for dealing with interpersonal conflict in the workplace: (1) begin from a place of curiosity and respect and don't worry about being liked, (2) focus on what you are hearing instead of formulating your response, (3) be direct, (4) don't put it off, and (5) expect a positive outcome. These techniques avoid creating further complications by framing the situation in a light that promotes open conversation and dialogue.

Conflicts of Party Interests

Although requesting clarification can help assess the meat of a problem between two employees or faculty members, more fact collection may be required for conflicts that originate not from a personal standpoint, but from an idealistic conflict, such as budgetary or policy-related conflicts, for example. It is imperative to gather all pertinent information to make decisions that benefit the most people.

Negotiation Strategies

Several negotiation strategies are useful for solving conflicts in the workplace. Because all conflicts are situation-based, and therefore inherently unique, there is no one size fits all strategy that can solve everything. Instead, it is the responsibility of a leader via mediation or facilitation to determine the best response to each situation as it comes. The first and most effective strategy is simply to problem-solve and find a resolution that satisfies the needs of every party involved. Although this course of action seems simple, execution can be much harder and altogether impossible in some cases. In the event that problem-solving of this nature is not feasible, try the alternative techniques described below.

Yielding to the Needs of Others

Sometimes, and especially during interpersonal conflicts, a team member may not have a problem of extensive or sophisticated origin. It may be easier to simply yield to the involved parties' requests. Before making the decision to yield, however, be sure to consider the weight of the action in terms of how each party will feel at the end, and whether the action may set a precedence. For example, yielding can be ineffective in situations that are particularly time-sensitive, such as absences or tardiness. It is important to avoid yielding excessively or out of convenience, as the original problems can reoccur.

Compromising with All Parties

Compromise if often thought of as the holy grail of conflict resolution. Although it is a highly effective technique, it is not a win-win resolution because all parties will only have their needs or interests partially met. Some needs or wants will have to be abandoned on both sides. In certain cases, there is no way to partially satisfy the needs of all parties, such as when purchasing lab equipment or when two professors vie for the same office space. However, compromise typically works well as a long-term solution. Parties are typically appeased enough to abide by the terms of the resolution. This technique is the closest to a win-win solution if there is no better option available.

Contending

Compromising and yielding are not always options for conflict resolution. There are instances where the needs of the department or company overshadow the wishes or interest of a single party. It can be uncomfortable to stand your ground, but it is sometimes necessary. It is important to be aware that if an attempt to contend is unsuccessful, it may be more difficult to use it in the future.

Inaction

Inaction is typically the last resort. Making the decision to do nothing in the short-term does allow more time to assess the situation in the long-term, though. In some cases, the conflict may diffuse altogether. Certain conflicts require nothing more than time to resolve them. Be careful to assess the depth of the situation before utilizing this technique—if the extent of a conflict is underestimated and a leader decides on inaction, a situation can easily escalate to a much bigger conflict than if it had been addressed initially. Inaction could also increase the time pressure to find later solutions.

Implementation and Evaluation

After the situation has been assessed and all possible responses have been given ample consideration, leaders must implement a plan of action. Several questions should be considered at this stage:

1. Does the problem require immediate action?
2. Would immediate action generate more problems or severely disrupt the workplace?
3. Is it feasible to implement a solution quickly in one stage, or would it be better to phase it in?

Some additional considerations are whether the conflict involves violations of the law or the ASHA Code of Ethics. Conflicts of this severity require immediate assessment and resolution. Additional support from superiors, attorneys, or law enforcement may be required.

Professional Issues of Power in the Field of Communication Science Disorders

The ASHA Leader addresses several modern issues related to power in the communication sciences and disorders field, such as the ramifications of speech-language disorders present within a practitioner in the field (Polovoy, Law, & Cutter, 2012).As stated previously, as professional (re)habilitators of communication there is some irony in the need for explicit instruction about communicative nuances among team members. Cynthia Clark in *The ASHA Leader* describes a healthy workplace environment as, "where mutual respect and professionalism carry the day, and faculty feel valued and supported by trustworthy, ethical, visionary leaders and rewarded for their contributions to the department and institution" (2017, p. 54). In another ASHA article, Law (2017) describes workplace hostility and strategies to overcome a hostile work environment that start at the ground level, with employees assisting in modifying unprofessional behaviors among staff before they escalate. Such tactics can include a "cup of coffee approach" to de-escalate or clarify issues in a nonthreatening manner and renew perspective within a department.

Incivility and Bullying

There is a very fine line between what constitutes incivility and what constitutes bullying, and effective leaders must recognize the effects of both in workplace environments. According to a study by the American Psychological Association (APA), workers in healthy workplace environments report "lower turnover (21% versus 40%) and high job satisfaction (91% versus 70%), and "are more motivated (44% versus 70%)," when compared to those in workplace environments with high rates of incivility and bullying (Clark, 2017, p. 58). The flip side of these statistics suggest several negative consequences of allowing incivility and bullying to flourish in a work environment.

Prevention is always the best strategy to avoid aversive behavior, but unfortunately, unless you are building a program or department from the ground up, this strategy is an unrealistic first step. Begin instead by dealing with the existing problem. Conduct an assessment of the current temperature of the work environment. The assessment should include leaders objectively evaluating themselves. "Seeking Civility Among Faculty" (Clark, 2017) suggests "to take an accurate inventory of your own behaviors and interactions and consider the impact they may have on others," (p. 57). Leaders' actions perceived more negatively than intended may simply be the result of miscommunication, as opposed to true malicious intent.

After completing a thorough assessment the question becomes, how do leaders eradicate and prevent future, aversive behaviors?

Action

The answer is that once problem behaviors are identified, leaders must make decisions and take action. Individual techniques for negotiation are covered later in the chapter, but for now, consider these strategies to remember:

1. Documentation is important. Include dates, times, and details of the aversive behaviors to promote accountability and mediate false perceptions of favoritism.
2. Do not put off dealing with difficult situations. The longer negative behavior exists, the more time it has to incubate and intensify. Hurt feelings based on perceived inequalities between workers can lead to incivility.
3. Provide specified and adequate avenues for employees to express their concerns. Creating an inclusive, open environment in the workplace is an active process. It requires maintenance, rather than a one-time fix. Open dialogue can fix misconceptions, and allow workers to consider all viewpoints, a major part of the definition of civility.

Leadership and Supervision in Academia

For leaders in academia, the development of competent clinicians necessitates additional supervisory nuances. Professors and other supervisors must facilitate the development of their students' hard and soft skills. Although this does require some tough love in certain instances, make sure that both you and the supervisors under you comprehend the difference between objective teaching and abusing the supervisory or professorial role.

ASHA created a committee in 2013 specifically tasked with outlining the supervisory role, and the findings of said commit-

tee are available on ASHA's website (http://www.asha.org/PRP
SpecificTopic.aspx?folderid=8589942113&section=Key_Issues).
The document specifies the five major pitfalls for clinical supervision: (1) halo effect, (2) central tendency, (3) similar-to-me effect,
(4) judgmental bias, and (5) leniency/strictness error (ASHA,
n.d.). Earlier generations of supervisors often used a much
harsher method of teaching than currently used, intended to
instill a strong core and sense of responsibility in new clinicians.
However, recent studies show that a more collaborative approach
benefits students more. *The ASHA Leader* recently published an
article on the effects of supervisors who abuse power, (Mancinelli, 2017). Along with describing psychological and physical
differences noticed in students, Mancinelli gives his professional
opinion on the perspective of students and field clinical educators (FCEs), or supervisors. He says, "bullying and intimidation
as a clinical teaching method has no place in the development
of the student's ability to think critically, solve problems, and
optimally treat the people we serve," (Mancinelli, 2017, p. 8).
It is then important to remember to actively listen to both the
students and the supervisors. Problems are almost never entirely
one-sided. Even though communication specialists are not therapists of the traditional variety, supervisors should be conscious
of any observed psychological or physical stress in their students
and other employees that may be work-related.

Application of Evidence-Based Practice

As scientifically oriented professionals, leaders in CSD should
always pursue avenues of best evidence-based practice. This
ideal should transfer to power and leadership dynamics as
well. When conflicts occur in student-supervisor and employer-
employee dynamics, prevention begins by consulting established
precedents and setting clear expectations between parties. If
problems arise later, there are already clear guidelines to resolve
the issues and immediately begin mediation. Signed agreements
as to what transpired and steps moving forward toward resolution are preferable purely for the sake of documentation and
accountability.

Addressing Conflict Specifically with Clinicians, Students, or Employees

When addressing conflicts involving student (or employee) performance, following some specific sequences can optimize the process of finding resolutions. Dr. Lemmon-Bush, undergraduate program director and clinical supervisor at Columbia College's Speech Language Pathology program, uses the sandwich method (Belludi, 2008) for her students. This route directly addresses the source of conflict, but surrounds that conflict with positivity, effectively sandwiching it, as described below.

Begin on a positive note by first highlighting work that a clinician, student or employee does well. This keeps the meeting from starting on a negative note and makes the clinician more likely to be open to constructive criticism. As per behavioral analysis theory, it effectively increases their behavior momentum (Skinner, 1938). After sharing some of the student's or employee's strengths, such as good client rapport or session flow, transition the conversation to the conflict at hand.

The conversation should always center on the action and not the person—this keeps the conversation professional and from sounding like a personal attack. In cases where the issue comes from a student or employee's demeanor, have clear and (hopefully) written expectations. It can be difficult to address such behavior without attacking a clinician's personality, but try to avoid that route, for two reasons. First, the criticism can cause further discord and future conflict between a supervisor and their student or employee. Second, a personal attack is unlikely to be received well or successfully incorporated in feedback. It is not the job of a leader to change the personality or demeanor of their subordinates except to the extent that it interferes with a person's ability to carry out their work duties.

Next, provide suggestions to fix the problem. It is far easier to point out problems than it is to find viable solutions. Be sure to have at least one idea or direction for improving unwanted behaviors. Providing choices increases cooperation between the supervisor and the student or employee. Providing choices gives students and employees the feeling of freedom, rather than feeling like they are being dictatorially ordered to fix a problem.

Be sure to end on a positive note. This note can come directly from the meeting itself, such as acknowledging a clinician's openness to improvement or appreciating a clinician making collaborative suggestions to fix the issue. The importance of leaving a student or employee with the hope to improve cannot be overstressed. The phrase, "there is always room for improvement," applies well in these types of situations. A sense of empowerment and personal accountability comes from approaching problems this way, leaving the person receiving criticism or feedback with the feeling that they are, in fact, capable of improvement.

Conclusion

Negotiation, conflict resolution, and workplace politics can be daunting for a leader, especially for leaders who are new to the role or to formal leadership in general. It is important for leaders to actively seek new evidence-based strategies, the input and assistance of both subordinates and superiors, and frequently self-assess their attitudes and actions. By gaining explicit knowledge of conflict resolution and strategies to nullify potentially harmful situations, leaders can increase the effectiveness and cohesiveness of their team. These approaches to leadership provide better feedback for leaders and better workplace satisfaction for team members.

Reflection

How is social power related to the concepts of effective leadership in academic and clinic environments? What are some sources of information on this topic and how can we begin to model these concepts in educational settings and professional settings?

References

ASHA. (n.d.). Clinical Education and Supervision: Key Issues. Retrieved from https://www.asha.org/PRPSpecificTopic.aspx?folderid=858994 2113&section=Key_Issues

Belludi, N. (2008). The compliment sandwich technique feedback technique, with examples. Retrieved from http://www.rightattitudes.com/2008/02/20/sandwich-feedback-technique/

Clark, C. (2017). Seeking civility among faculty. *The ASHA Leader*, *22*(12), 54–59. https://doi.org/10.1044/leader.FTR2.22122017.54

Duggan, T. (n.d.). Problem solving skills training & the workplace [Online newspaper article]. *Chron.com*. Retrieved from http://small business.chron.com/problem-solving-skills-training-workplace-116 56.html

Garfinkle, J. (2017, May 24). How to have difficult conversations when you don't like conflict. *Harvard Business Review*. Retrieved from https://hbr.org/2017/05/how-to-have-difficult-conversations-when-you-dont-like-conflict

Law, B. M. (2017). That's just mean. *The ASHA Leader*, *22*(12), 46–53. https://doi.org/10.1044/leader.FTR1.22122017.46

Mancinelli, J. M. (2017). Bullying and intimidation in clinical supervision. *The ASHA Leader*, *22*(12), 8–10. https://doi.org/10.1044/leader.FMP.22122017.8

Natter, E.. (2018, June 29. 5 Types of Power in Businesses [Online newspaper article]. *Chron.com*. Retrieved from http://smallbusiness.chron.com/5-types-power-businesses-18221.html

Polovoy, C., Law, B. M., & Cutter, M. (2012). Motivated by their struggles. *The AHSA Leader,* 17(6), 16-19. doi.org/10.1044/leader.FTR2.17062012.16

Skinner, B. F. (1938). *The Behavior of organisms: An experimental analysis*. New York, NY: Appleton-Century.

8

Leadership Wellness: Establishing Healthy Leadership Cultures

Wendy Papir-Bernstein

The ability to work, the desire to work, the ability to maintain work and to apply yourself in work, while preserving part of your life, attention and energy for greater endeavors and studies, represents a mature and successful approach in building this pillar of your foundation.

—Marshall Vian Summers

Learning Objectives

- Readers will learn about the importance of well-being and self-care as they relate to the creation of healthy organizational cultures.
- Readers will learn about branding and professional advocacy as components of leadership wellness.
- Readers will learn about the impact of professional impairment and burnout on the work environment, and learn about strategies for buffering stress.

- Readers will learn about assessing the internal communications environment for the purpose of creating a collaborative leadership culture within a dynamic learning environment.

Introduction

As leaders in our field, prescriptions for our own self-care and well-being must be at least as important as care for the people who work within our organizations, our hospitals, our universities, our communities, and our school settings. *Self-care* refers to attitudes and actions that contribute to the maintenance of well-being. It is not about having an emergency response plan or a list of things to do, and it need not lead to feelings of selfishness. Rather, leadership well-being demands mindful attention to our daily activities, and identification of situations that become stressful.

Well-Being

As leaders, we must examine our personal attitudes about well-being before we begin to consider the well-being of our organization. Our work reflects our personal attitudes about our own well-being, as much as about the well-being of our patients, clients, and students. In fact, our personal attitudes are an integral component of clinical expertise and will drive the success of our practice and leadership programs. It is not surprising that the description of personal attitudes and qualities has recently been expanded in both ASHA's 2014 clinical competency standards as *interaction and personal qualities*, and in the 2015 revision of standards for accreditation of graduate programs as *professional practice competencies* (ASHA, 2014a, 2015a). Attitudes provide a framework and context for what happens within clinical and educational processes, and are thus the most critical tool in the profession (Papir-Bernstein, 2018).

Well-being is sometimes linked to Aristotle's idea of *eudaimonia*, the belief that the overarching goal of all human actions is to flourish (Bradburn, 1969). Well-being has been compared to quality of life, defined by the World Health Organization (WHO) as "an individual's perception of their position in life in the context of the culture and value systems in which they live in relation to their goals, expectations, standards and concerns" (World Health Organization [WHO], 1997, p. 1). Martin Seligman, a leader in the positive psychology movement, developed a theory about the building blocks for a life that flourishes, for which he coined the term PERMA: positive emotion, engagement, relationships, meaning, and accomplishment (Papir-Bernstein, 2018; Seligman, 2011). Haidt, another researcher from the field of positive psychology, tells us that well-being and happiness, whether personal or professional, are driven by the same themes: we want to make a difference, we want to be useful, we want to connect with something greater than ourselves, we want balance in our lives, and we want community (Haidt, 2006).

Each us has our own individual set point for well-being. It exists on a kind of seesaw, impacted by resources on one side and challenges on the other. In the work setting, when challenges affect the fluctuating state of our well-being equilibrium and create an imbalance, we need to adapt our resources to meet the challenge. One resource is the ability to use perspective to reframe events. Well-being is difficult to define and measure; however, many of us have experienced that equilibrium is easily offset by life's challenges. Sometimes we link well-being to success in terms of how much we contribute to the quality of our own lives and the lives of others (Papir-Bernstein, 2018). How do we measure such success? We are familiar with the measures used for client outcomes, but how do we measure our own contributions, which enhance our lives and the lives of our clients? Arianna Huffington talks about using a metric that extends beyond money and power. She calls it *meaning* (Huffington, 2015). The meaning metric shifts the measurement from external to internal. When we use meaning as a metric of success, we create opportunity for reflection and self-direction.

Marketing and Branding

Marketing and branding is an important component of leadership wellness. We work in a service profession, whether educationally or medically based. At some point in our careers, we need to market our services, our philosophy, or our use of specific materials and methodologies. Marketing involves telling potential clients why your practice or organization is the best (Polovoy, 2015). As we think about our marketing strategies, we also need to think about positioning and branding.

Branding relates to internal organizational philosophies and the context of messages to audiences external to the organization where you work. How do you know if your organization needs to develop a branding philosophy? Sometimes branding statements are implicit within the organizational structure; but everyone in the organization needs to deliver the same simple message. Your brand must not be a secret. All organizations need coherent brand ideas that guide purposeful strategies. Your brand is essential for cultivating a positive perception of your services in the marketplace.

The 2012 ASHA Changing Healthcare Landscape Summit ([CHLS]; ASHA CHLS, 2012) began a dialogue about the importance of branding and rebranding. in our rapidly changing health care landscape and the impact of the rapid changes on the field. As is commonly acknowledged, the primary role of our national association is to safeguard the professions in light of disruptions and evolution to our existing landscape. A prominent topic at the summit was the reframing or rebranding of our professions as the *leaders in communication health*. For example, one suggestion was to change the vocabulary used to describe *value* to person-centered rather than disability-centered—in our assessments, intervention, and reporting of outcomes.

At the 2017 ASHA convention in Los Angeles, the theme of branding was once again picked up for discussion. ASHA set up what they called an empowerment zone to enable students and working professionals to sharpen their personal advocacy skills by learning about personal branding and its relationship to the development of leadership skills. Personal branding facilitates awareness of how individuals' profiles can impact the perception of our training and skills within our social and professional communities.

Singletary and Smith (2014) developed suggestions for how to incorporate branding into messages and materials that can be used for a variety of purposes, including recruitment of subjects into clinical trials and personnel recruitment. As materials are developed, we need to be sure they have a consistent look and feel. Organizational materials might include talking points, fact sheets, and articles and presentations with which the organization is involved. Logos are another way to communicate your brand (Michael J. Fox Foundation [MJFF], 2014). For example, ASHA has a specific "brand block" that is used for all ASHA approved CE providers. Another consideration is development of a solid *positioning statement.* Positioning statements consider segments of the market and potential clients, and will differ depending on the clients you are trying to attract (Polovoy, 2015).

James Heaton of Tronvig Group (2016) presents a brand pyramid as a series of questions used as a benchmark to measure the impact of branding ideas and check their alignment with your organization and its members. Everyone needs to be on the same page.

- Features and attributes: What are the attributes of your brand?
- Tangible benefits: What are the specific functional benefits and unique features delivered to consumers, compared to other brands?
- Emotional benefits: Why do your consumers care about working with you in particular?
- Brand personality: What values underlie your specific brand?
- Brand essence: Does your brand continue to exist outside of your "brand bubble," or organization?

Another strategy to facilitate branding is developing an elevator speech. *Elevator speeches* are sometime the ideal platform for introducing a brand, marketing an idea, selling a solution, or simply raising awareness of an issue. They are generally around 3 minutes, the time it takes for people in an elevator to travel from the top floor to the bottom. The term originally came into play in Hollywood, when screenwriters had limited time to pitch ideas to a producer so they had to be ready at a moment's notice.

Often, an elevator speech gets the ball rolling by beginning a dialogue that needs to be continued, or introduces an idea that needs to be researched and further considered. Every word is carefully planned and chosen, and the speech should contain four components: an introduction, body, conclusion, and call to action. The *introduction* captures the attention of the listener and informs the listener of what to expect. The *body of the speech* should have no more than three talking points. The *conclusion* should be a summary of those main points, and allude to what discussion needs to be continued in the future. Finally, the *call to action* is the request you are making of the listener, such as an email, meeting or phone call. Nine Cs have been proposed as necessary for success: the pitch should be concise, clear, credible, compelling, concrete, conceptual, consistent, conversational, and customized. In summary, elevator speeches should contain careful consideration of personal vocal styles, body language, charisma, authenticity, creativity, and timing (Ellis, Gottfred, & Freiberg, 2015; Papir-Bernstein, 2018; Sjodin, 2012).

Professional Advocacy

Advocacy is another important component of leadership wellness. Without it, we miss out on funding and support. Admittedly, we work in an interconnected world and have easier access than ever before to public policy legislative issues and the people who move them into laws. *Legislative, or grassroots advocacy,* involves the identification of key issues and the individuals and associations that work together to facilitate either the passing of or prevention of legislation (Ruder, Noplock, & Johnson, 2003). Advocacy encompasses a broad range of activities conducted to influence decision-makers at various levels, including not only traditional advocacy work such as lobbying, but also capacity building, network formation, relationship building, communication, and leadership development. Most professionals who consider themselves advocates rarely devote 100% of their time and resources to advocacy efforts; they are usually involved with primary businesses devoted to direct service activities (Gardner & Brindis, 2017; Wright & Wright, 2016).

Some of the best research studies from advocacy networks evolve out of the nonprofit sector, as those organizations rely on advocacy and policy change efforts to drive public and private funding to their programs. A study commissioned by the Annie E. Casey Foundation for Innovation Network (Inovation Network [IN], 2008), surveyed 200 participants from across the nonprofit advocacy sector to develop practical recommendations for implementing and evaluating advocacy efforts. Results showed that the first step is increasing awareness of the need for action; the second step is developing methodologies, tools, and program strategies to improve advocacy activities; and the third step is developing evaluation practices for whatever advocacy activities take place (Sue & Ritter, 2007).

The Innovation Network study reported that only one in four organizations evaluated its advocacy work to demonstrate the impact their advocacy efforts. Two simple, open-ended questions for reflection on organizational advocacy effectiveness are as follows: (1) Which advocacy activities are used by your organization? (2) Which of those activities have been most effective, and why? *Advocacy capacity building* refers to activities that strengthen an organization's ability to effectively sustain advocacy efforts. Examples might include educating the public, networking with other organizations, and organizing constituency groups. Organizational capacity for advocacy can be measured with indicators such as decision-making structures, organizational commitment to advocacy, resources for advocacy, and knowledge and systems in place to implement advocacy strategies. *Education and awareness building* (related to branding and marketing) includes research, media outreach, public events, website development, and newsletters.

In that same study, the most effective strategies used for advocacy by organizations cited in the study included education (59%), community or grassroots organizing (47%), and coalition building through civic and community engagement (26%; IN, 2008). Grassroots action and coalition building have unique power to influence policymakers. Partnering with allies facilitates a stronger and more credible voice to pursue policy change.

Advocacy teams often work in concert with association lobbyists. Why do we need lobbyists? Simply put, practitioners have neither the time to commute to the state capital on a regular basis, nor the familiarity with all the intricacies of the legislative process. Lobbyists walk legislative halls on a regular basis, and understand the issues and the personal and professional circumstances that might influence an individual to support your issue. This legislative individual is sometimes called *the champion*, and is targeted for one or more of the following reasons (Henri, 2011):

1. They are familiar with the issue you are addressing because they or a family member have had personal experience with it.
2. They hold a leadership position, such as head of the finance committee in the House or Senate.
3. They have collaborated with other legislators working on similar issues.
4. They have collaborated with either you or your lobbyist on similar issues.

There are many resources that our national and state associations make available so that we can be better informed and perhaps launch successful advocacy campaigns. ASHA's advocacy portal contains news about the latest legislative actions, a member advocacy section, the Public Policy Agenda, links to information about your state, related to regulations and contacts, and additional advocacy resources. For example, if you click on "Take Action," all of the trending issues appear, with information sheets you can download and sample language to help you write letters of support to your legislative representatives to advocate for specific bills. It couldn't be any easier to get involved. There are currently six ASHA staff members who work on federal advocacy, political advocacy, educational advocacy, regulatory advocacy, congressional advocacy, and grassroots member engagement (ASHA Advocacy, State Advocacy). It is imperative to remember that by supporting your national and state associations, you support the profession and sustain the field by modeling leadership practices for those who follow. Nothing speaks to advocacy louder than volunteer leadership work, which will be discussed in more detail when we talk about leadership trends in the following chapter.

Professional Impairment and Burnout

As leaders in our field, one of our responsibilities is to recognize symptoms of potential burnout and develop organizational and personal strategies for combating stress. Burnout often begins with symptoms of professional impairment. One of the most complete definitions of professional impairment comes from the American Medical Association. It is as attributed to a practitioner who is unable to practice with skill and safety due to physical or mental illness, deterioration through the aging process or motor dysfunction, personal or family problems that interfere with the quality or care and interpersonal communication, or substance abuse. This is a potential issue with all practitioners and leaders involved with communication sciences, education, and health care (Pfifferling, 1986).

It is no surprise that when job satisfaction is low and retention rates dip, two of the major contributors are stress and burnout (Ross, 2011). Stress is caused by external as well as internal factors, such as decreased hope, increased fear, and mismatched beliefs and expectations. Studies show that some of the more common work stressors are paperwork, tension in relationships, attitudes of competitiveness, conflicting values, poor teaming, overcommitment, lack of physical relaxation, and lack of time to complete work (Felt, 2014; Flasher & Fogle, 2012).

In demanding situations, a stress response may or may not occur depending on the balance arising from the interaction of external demands, internal values, personal coping strategies, and external resources and support. The four most common reasons we experience our work as inherently stressful are: the complexity of our client base, the difficulty of experiencing outcomes, poor perceptions of relationships, and frustration with the systematic decision-making process. In essence, our work becomes more tedious and less rewarding (Lubinski & Hudson, 2013; Papir-Bernstein, 2018).

Burnout is a state of physical, emotional, spiritual and/or mental exhaustion resulting from poor coping strategies, in conjunction with involvement with people and situations that are emotionally demanding (Pines, 1986). It is caused by and results in an erosion of engagement. Pines and Aronson (1988) conducted over a decade of research with more than 5,000 human service professionals from more than 25 occupations in seven countries. The conceptual framework for the research was a social-psychological model that assumes most human service professionals start their careers with high levels of motivation. The research found that when we work in a supportive environment and achieve peak performance, motivation gets reinforced and strengthened and becomes self-sustaining. Professional burnout occurs when demands increase and resources fail to keep pace, or when personal values and organizational values are in a state of discord (Papir-Bernstein, 2018).

Burnout can be experienced as the final stage of stress, and has been described as emotional exhaustion, depersonalization, and reduced feelings of personal accomplishment. In professions such as ours, burnout has been termed *compassion fatigue* because of the emotional demands of caring for people along with our inability to cope with environmental demands. Compassion fatigue is a psychological and emotional state that depletes motivation and energy, sometimes resulting in anger, hostility and irritability with friends, family, and coworkers (LaRowe, 2008).

There are three recognized stages of burnout: stress arousal, energy conservation, and exhaustion. *Stress arousal* includes physiological and psychological responses characterized by gastrointestinal disorders, headaches, irritability, anxiety, and forgetfulness. In the *energy conservation* phase, individuals attempt to compensate for stress with lateness, procrastination leading to missed deadlines, excessive time off, and unusual fatigue. It is only in the final stage of burnout, *exhaustion*, where professionals get a sense that something is wrong. Symptoms may include chronic gastrointestinal problems or headaches, chronic sadness or depression, and social isolation (Lubinski & Hudson, 2013; Papir-Bernstein, 2018; Ross, 2011; Texas Medical Association, 2010).

Symptoms of burnout have been categorized as physical, affective-cognitive, and behavioral. In addition to the symptoms already mentioned, burned out professionals can also experience emotional exhaustion, depersonalization, and a reduced sense of accomplishment. Behaviors reported in our field include frequent irritation or increased moodiness, more frequent illness caused by lowered immunity, difficulty focusing, decreased motivation to engage in new projects, and little optimism about work population and setting (Flasher & Fogle, 2012; Langdon & Langdon Starr, 2014). Hale, Kellum, and Burger (2006) reported a positive correlation between lower stress levels and the utilization of coping mechanisms such as humor, laughter, and friendships in the workplace. However, when faced with stressful situations, and either the presence of negative features (exhaustion) or absence of positive features (support), burnout may be the result. Ultimately, the determining factor in whether an individual will reach peak performance or burn out is the balance between personal dispositional characteristics and the work environment (Papir-Bernstein, 2018).

Research in the area of human service provision indicates that the tendency for burnout in that community of workers is high for two reasons: the interpersonal nature of the work, and the organizational factors that often arise in social, educational, and health care agencies. In a meta-analysis of 35 years of research about burnout, Schaufeli, Leiter, and Maslach (2009) concluded that developments in science, like the emergence of positive psychology, coupled with focus on organizational behaviors, can impact work engagement and lead to a decrease in burnout behaviors. Whereas burnout is viewed as the negative pole on a continuum of employee well-being, work engagement constitutes the opposite, positive pole. Work engagement includes communication strategies for giving and receiving social support, and maintaining a sense of community (Pines, 1982; Scott, 2007).

The Impact of Work Environment on Stress and Burnout

Creating healthier physical and social environments to support employee health and safety is part of a leader's role. Leaders are gatekeepers who often allocate resources to create conditions conducive to successful outcomes for members of the workplace community (Human Resources Institute [HRI], 2011). The development of wellness leaders is gaining popularity in wellness program design with the knowledge that leaders play a central role in creating effective programs. This is a big departure from a primary focus on individual outreach and education by experts outside of an organization. The newer model involves organizational resources that support individual change (Allen, 2008).

Pines and Aronson (1988) identified dimensions and features of supportive work environments, as distinguished from stressful work environments. They describe a number of variables that play a role in promoting or preventing burnout, represented by four dimensions of the environment: psychological, physical, social and organizational. Supportive work environments have the positive features of autonomy, variety, actualization, significance, growth, support, and challenge. Stressful work environments have the negative features of overload, noise, bureaucratic red tape, paperwork, and communication problems. Although some work factors relative to our environments are under our influence, others are not. We must learn to recognize factors that work for us and those that do not, choose carefully, and exert leadership to navigate changes in the work environment when necessary (Papir-Bernstein, 2018).

Psychological dimensions include emotional and cognitive variables. One of the emotional variable that accounts for job dissatisfaction is the belief that our work has no real significance. Some jobs feel inherently more important than others, but work environments can enhance or diminish how individuals perceived the significance of their work. In our work, the best way to feel our impact is through the outcomes that our clients achieve. A second emotional variable is the need for actualization and growth, which according to Maslow (1968) is at the highest point in our hierarchy of needs. *Self-actualization* refers to the need for personal growth and discovery that remains present throughout life.

The *cognitive variables* of the psychological dimension include autonomy, variety, and overload. A sense of autonomy ties in with a need for power and control, both of which work against stress as they help us feel that we can predict and determine what will happen in our immediate environment. Autonomy is a high predictor of job satisfaction. Variety, too, can enhance job satisfaction, job performance, and simply showing up for work. Most people actively seek variety and avoid monotonous situations. Variety enhances interest and challenge. *Overload* occurs when individuals' have too many tasks to complete, or tasks that are too difficult (Papir-Bernstein, 2018).

Social dimensions of the work environment include the people with whom we work and our relationships with them and with service recipients (and the challenges that ensue). *Organizational dimensions* target bureaucratic red tape, rules and regulations, and policy influence (and role conflicts that ensue). *Physical dimensions* include architectural structure, space, noise, and the amount of flexibility we have to change fixed features.

There is a growing body of evidence that physical dimensions of our environment impact our mental and physical health, and that area of study is now called *environmental psychology*. From an environmental psychology perspective, stress has been defined as a mismatch between an individual's needs and the attributes of their environment. If workers are fortunate enough to have their own space at work, that space is probably far from ideal. We can throw up our hands and complain or be proactive about making it the best space that it can possibly be. Some elements that can be fixed are more obvious than others, like clutter, heat, and light. We can learn about other spatial elements by examining some basic design principles used by feng shui practitioners to harmonize people with their surrounding environment. Alignment and balance are the essence of this ancient Chinese design art, and the first step is to heighten your awareness of the space. There may be some easy fixes incorporating shapes, materials, colors, objects and their locations, and orientation of furniture. (Papir-Bernstein, 2018; Skinner, 2001).

One additional area of potential stress and burnout that is very much in the news today and deserves mention is civility, and the lack thereof in the workplace. A healthy work environment is one in which workers can thrive because they feel respected, valued, supported, and rewarded. On the other hand, bullying, demeaning behaviors, condescending attitudes, and disparaging remarks contribute to an unhealthy environment. Business leadership programs have been revising syllabuses because bad behavior by big companies has led the front page of newspapers to be plastered with stories about ethics. Our understanding of ethics and values and the part they play in leadership has recently been challenged in public media and pop culture. Bottom-line business training programs are drawing more content than ever before from social sciences rather than from the financial world, include topics such as empathy and communications (Gelles & Miller, 2017).

A 2016 Civility in America study reported that 75% of respondents believed incivility had risen to crisis levels, and 84% of workers had experienced incivility at work (Clark, 2017). Following are some suggestions for fostering civility, beginning with your own behavior, as a leader within your own organization:

1. Reflect on your own behaviors and interactions and consider the impact they have on others.
2. Define desirable and undesirable behaviors.
3. Determine consequences of problematic behaviors.
4. Attend to your own physical, emotional and spiritual wellness.

Individual Strategies for Managing Stress

During times of stress we become more reactive and less proactive. We tend to resist, blame, compete, justify, suspect, and struggle. Transforming a downward spiral into a cycle of growth is entirely possible, as long as we reflect and rebalance. LaRowe (2008) outlines three principles essential for healing and transformation: self-honesty, personal responsibility, and self-expression. All of these principles involves transparency, insight and reflection. They are skillful concepts that can be facilitated and learned through a willingness to take ownership of personal experiences, perspectives, thoughts, and emotions.

In their book about impaired physicians and physicians-in-training, Scott and Hawk (1986) coined the term *compleat physician* with the Old English spelling to emphasize the word "complete." Compleat physicians understand that sensitivity and technical competence are important to patient care, and make an effort to understand and implement these qualities in their own lives. They nurture affective qualities, and are not been swept along by social forces that promote career attainment at the expense of personal and family well-being. It can be argued that *impaired* and *compleat* are idealized terms, and that many individuals vary in degree between the two. However, the movement in one direction or another is a "developmental process, not a cataclysmic event" and reflects the fact that professional careers are dynamic in nature (Scott & Hawk, 1986).

Ross (2011) explains that strategies for stress management and burnout avoidance include cognitive, emotional, social, spiritual-philosophical, and physical dimensions. Cognitive, intellectual and mental strategies begin with knowledge of what constitutes burnout, followed by activities like desensitization, problem-setting, and reframing. Emotional strategies include promoting self-awareness, consultations, recalibrating goals, and incorporating time-outs and work breaks. Social strategies include reaching out for support from other professionals, friends and family; engaging in morale building activities; and balancing work and home life. Spiritual-philosophical strategies include activities to foster renewal and mindfulness. Physical strategies include exercise, rest, and anything done for relaxation (Papir-Bernstein, 2018).

Langdon and Langdon Starr (2014) offer suggestions for nurturing your mind, body, spirit, and emotions. Nurture your mind by being reflective and self-aware, taking breaks, creating and developing new methods and materials, and scheduling in fun. Nurture your body by walking during work breaks, sticking to a healthy diet, and considering brief shoulder and chair massages. These suggestions are especially important for professionals who spend a lot of time sitting. Nurture your spirit by focusing on your strengths, staying away from negative people and gossip, looking for coworkers who share your perspectives, and scheduling in a change of scenery. Nurture your emotions by facilitating positive relationships, consulting with colleagues, and talking with family members or professionals if you need additional support (Papir-Bernstein, 2018).

In essence, the management of stress is a dynamic process that involves our emotional, physical, cognitive, social, and spiritual ways of thinking, feeling, and being. It involves ongoing reflection, self-assessment, and rebalance. Felt (2014) identifies a number of steps in this process of rebalancing ourselves (Papir-Bernstein, 2018):

1. Stop and reflect: Ask yourself "what do I love to do?, what are my gifts?, what are my passions?, what are my beliefs, what do I really enjoy?"
2. Look: Assess where you are in all areas of your life. Are there some other areas that need attention? Consider finances, your home, friends and family, fitness and health, significant others, and leisure.
3. Choose: Have you chosen to devote more attention to some areas of your life to the detriment of others? Are you choosing to get drawn into ego and political battles?
4. Re-establish goals: Draw a map of where you would like to be, and plan out the steps you need to accomplish to get there. Use the SMART system for your goals: be specific, measurable, attainable, realistic, and on a timetable. Track and measure your progress.
5. Acknowledge yourself: Solicit positive feedback, and give it to yourself as well. Celebrate your victories and have fun along the way.

Organizational Strategies for Buffering Stress and Burnout Potential

One major organizational strategy that buffers the potential for individual burnout is social support. *Social support* is defined as any type of information or action that leads individuals to believe they are valued within the network of communications and mutual agreements. Prescriptive models for workplace communications tend to be holistic and include qualities such as supportiveness, trust and confidence, credibility, and openness and candor in message sending and receiving (Cobb, 1976; Redding, 1972). Workplace communication will be discussed in more detail later in the chapter.

Pines and Aronson (1988) grouped supportive actions into six categories: listening, emotional support, emotional challenge, technical support, technical challenge, and sharing social reality. The support categories were based on dynamic communication exchanges that included expressions of appreciation, encouragement, and reinforcement, especially during times of technical and emotional challenge. Although leaders and managers could often name these strategies when surveyed, workers reported that they were underutilized. Scott's later research (2007) indicated that coworker interactions can reduce or increase burnout depending on other supports that may be in place, including participation in decision-making and perceptions of personal accomplishment.

Another organizational strategy is to establish some type of wellness program. About 20 years ago, the Wellness Councils of America collaborated with the Human Resources Institute (HRI) to investigate the role of organizational leaders in promoting wellness programs. The study revealed four leadership strategies that facilitate organizational wellness (Allen, Hunnicutt, & Johnson, 1999):

1. Sharing a wellness vision includes participating in the creation of organizational definitions, organizational strategies, and employee initiatives. Leaders support wellness programs by explaining how they work, why they are important, and how people can participate. A wellness vision needs to have a story rooted in the organization's history and tied to its hopes for the future.

2. Serving as a wellness role model by having balanced lifestyle and healthy habits. At a minimum, leaders should develop strategies for "walking the wellness talk," and should lower visibility of unhealthy habits and behaviors.

3. Implementing wellness touch points includes formal and informal cultural policies, communications, and training that influence health behaviors. Leaders often research wellness practices that found to be successful in similar organizations.

4. Monitoring and celebrating wellness success means insuring that individual and group wellness goals are set, measured, recognized, and rewarded. When it comes to rewards, financial incentives are not always

possible. Therefore, rewards also come in the form of praise, increased autonomy, access to resources, and choice of job responsibilities.

In summary, leadership advocacy and support for organizational wellness is a philosophy that needs to be stated, formalized, evaluated, and rewarded. Please see Appendix 8–A for one example of an organizational leadership wellness assessment.

Facilitating Knowledge—Sharing Cultures

Healthy organizations strive for ongoing integration of new information and expansion of the knowledge base. Today especially, we have unlimited access to information about any subject. Nate Silver reminds us that information is no longer a scarce commodity, and that we have more than we know what to do with. "We think we want information when we really want knowledge. Which is the signal, and which is the noise? The signal is the truth. The noise is what distracts us from the truth" (Silver, 2012, p. 17). Leaders ask, what is our truth, and what detracts us from seeing it? Where does our present fit into our past and future? What do we do with all of this information, and how do we make it work for us, our organization, and the people we serve (Papir-Bernstein, 2018)?

Organizational knowledge must be translated and presented so that the values of the organization are upheld and its mission is accomplished. One of the greatest challenges for leaders in any field is the building of meaningful learning experiences. O'Dell and Grayson (1988) said it best: we need to "get the right knowledge to the right people at the right time, and help people share and put information into action in ways that strive to improve organizational performance" (p. 6). Knowledge management strategists Gupta and Sharma (2004) list the most popular organizational strategies used across occupational fields as websites, communities of practice (CoP), social learning networks, storytelling, expert directories, knowledge fairs, mentors, knowledge repositories, cross-project learning, and after-action reviews, and debriefing sessions (Papir-Bernstein, 2018).

Many terms are used and systems of classification are devised to classify knowledge types. One of the most useful for our purposes is a knowledge framework that distinguishes between tacit, or personal knowledge and explicit, or formal knowledge. Whereas tacit elements are subjective and experiential, explicit elements are objective and rational. Tacit knowledge, which is often uncodified, comes from people's experiences and memories. It is best communicated through shared or described experiences. Tacit knowledge is deeply personal, reflecting perceptions, insights, and know-how (O'Dell & Grayson, 1998), as opposed to know-what (the facts), know-why (the science), or know-who (the networking; Papir-Bernstein, 2012). Explicit knowledge, usually more easily codified, can come from books, papers, written media, and policy manuals. Most explicit knowledge is technical and academic. It includes information that is formally shared through teaching and in textbooks, and requires a level of academic understanding acquired through formal education and structured study. The vast majority of information shared through our academic culture is formal, technical, and explicit.

Nonaka and Hirotaka (1995) said that learning is created at the intersection between tacit knowledge and explicit knowledge and describe a detailed relationship between the two systems. Whereas both tacit and explicit knowledge are valuable to any organization, one of the most vital of a leader's responsibilities is to protect and enhance sources of tacit knowledge by creating a culture of knowledge sharing, knowledge exchanges, and knowledge conversion (Papir-Bernstein, 2012). The sharing of tacit knowledge can take place only through physical proximity, like engaging in and interpersonal interactions and joint activities. Sharing tacit knowledge proceeds through four stages: socialization, externalization, combination, and internalization (Nonaka, 1994; Papir-Bernstein, 2018).

Socialization, sometimes referred to as brainstorming, is the first step, and transfers tacit knowledge between individuals through observation, imitation, and practice. *Externalization* means translating tacit knowledge into explicit procedures and documents via dialogue, reflections, and the use of analogy and metaphor. *Combination* reconfigures explicit knowledge by sorting, categorizing, and integrating information, and spreading it throughout the organization. This is sometimes referred to as best practices. *Internalization* is the final step, and links explicit knowledge with individuals' tacit knowledge, and thus, knowledge creation and sharing become part of the organization's culture.

After tacit knowledge is shared, it needs to be integrated with more explicit mediums. This is challenging because the knowledge sources are often so diverse. Tacit knowledge tends to involve more creative and insightful thinking, whereas explicit knowledge is logical and fact based. Therefore, explicit knowledge is more easily shared through formal structures, and tacit knowledge through storytelling, narratives, and use of metaphors.

Nonika (1994) and Smith (2001) describe four patterns of knowledge integration used in a variety of organizational structures (Papir-Bernstein, 2012, 2018). First, we move knowledge from tacit to tacit, as we learn from mentors and peers by observing, imitating and practicing with others. Second, we move knowledge from explicit to explicit, as we transform one type of explicit knowledge into another, like using data to generate reports. Third, we move knowledge from tacit to explicit, as we incorporate brainstorming discussions and innovations into a manual or other product. Fourth, we move knowledge from explicit to tacit, as we reframe our own perspective.

The following strategies for organizational knowledge sharing come from a variety of business and social science disciplines (Papir-Bernstein, 2018; Smith, 2001):

- Instill a corporate-wide culture that integrates knowledge resources into every organizational process.
- Support interactive learning experiences, and give and take communication.
- Encourage knowledge sharing by connecting people with varied expertise in content topic or geography with each other.
- Create idea bulletin boards.
- Implement CoP.
- Organize a talent exchange.
- Use extraordinary recruitment methods to attract, hire, and retain the most motivated and knowledgeable people.
- Create peer-to-peer networks.

Creation of Collaborative Learning Environments

This section discusses the importance of acknowledging expertise and creating collaborative cultures. The aggressive pursuit of lifelong learning must be an organizational priority, and speaks to the dynamic nature of our scope of practice and commitment to the people we serve. Organizational wellness will be reflected through our passionate devotion to professional development approaches.

Fullan (1990) posited that all learning is predicated on four cornerstones. First, we learn by doing and by evaluating and modifying information and actions. Second, we learn by connecting new information with prior information. Third, we learn by reflecting and monitoring our interpretations, behaviors, and decisions. Last, we learn by being in a supporting environment, and incorporating feedback that acknowledges our individual style and experience. In 1990 Peter Senge, founding chair of the Society for Organizational Learning (SoL), popularized the concept of *the learning organization* as an organization within which both individual and collective learning take place. Senge stressed the importance of organizations learning from the wisdom of its personnel by incorporating their insights to generate new ones. According to his definition, "the learning organization is an organization that possesses not only inductive capacity but also a generative one—that is the ability to create alternative future" (Senge, 2006, p. 14).

A learning organization can be described as the sum of individual learning for the good of the organization, but there must be vehicles in place for individual learning to transfer to organizational learning (Papir-Bernstein & Legrand, 1993; Papir-Bernstein, 2018). In his 2006 book *The Fifth Discipline*, Senge identified two features that learning organizations seem to have in common: personal mastery and shared learning. *Personal mastery* is seen as a commitment to the process of learning through the discipline of clarifying and deepening personal vision. This goes beyond competence and skills, but certainly involves both. Mastery is a lifelong process and a type of calling rather than simply a good idea suggested by the organization. Professionals with personal mastery are often deeply self-confident and may be perceived as a threat to an organization if individuals do not engage with a shared vision. Individual learning must be encouraged and valued in an environment where individuals can share what they have learned (Papir-Bernstein, 1995, 2018; Smith, 2001).

Every experience is as an opportunity to learn. In learning organizations, members are on a continuous learning track for the good of the organization and for their own individual professional growth. According to Kerka (1995), learning organizations function best when learning is continuous, valued, and shared. Learning organizations do the following (Papir-Bernstein, 2018; Senge, 2006):

1. Link individual performance with organizational performance
2. Make it safe for individuals to openly share
3. Embrace creative tension as a source of motivation, energy and transformation
4. Provide continuous learning opportunities
5. Use learning to facilitate their mission and vision

Both individual and shared learning are key reciprocal components of organizational wellness. The development of a shared vision provides motivation for all levels of staff, generates a focus and common energy for learning, and creates a common identity (Senge, 2006). Team or shared learning facilitates learning in individuals, just as individual learning contributes to team learning. With team learning, teams improves problem-solving capacity through better access to knowledge and expertise. The presence of organizational structures, such as open and easily crossed boundaries, facilitates team learning within learning organizations (Papir-Bernstein, 2018).

Earlier in the chapter we talked about how social supports, collaborations, networks, and CoP act as buffers to potential burnout. One type of community organized for the purpose of mutual learning is called a *professional learning community* (PLC). PLCs generally contain four components: shared beliefs, values and vision and a commitment to focus on organizational learning; shared and supportive leadership, including shared authority for decision-making; collective thinking and learning that lead to creative solutions; and shared personal practice, including comfort with sharing reflections and receiving feedback (Clark & Flynn, 2011; Papir-Bernstein, 2018; Rudebusch & Wiechmann, 2013).

Research has identified the following positive outcomes for administrators and support staff, such as speech-language pathologists, engagement in learning communities (Rudebusch & Wiechmann, 2013):

1. Greater commitment to the organization's mission and vision
2. Shared responsibility for outcomes
3. Reduced isolation
4. Increased understanding of content provided by all professionals
5. Higher morale and lower stress
6. Increased appreciation of role differentiation and professional expertise

Collaborations with members of professional learning communities allow us to take advantage of the expertise that we can only gain by crossing through the boundaries of individual perspectives and lines of professional disciplines. As we learn from one another, share skills and build team consensus, we extend our organizational functions beyond a knowledge-based or political hierarchy (Papir-Bernstein, 2018; Pickering & Embry, 2013). Personal learning communities are sometimes referred to as *social learning environments*.

Social learning focuses on learning in organizational settings through relationships with others and engaging in actual situations of practice with observation and authentic participation in CoP (Harris, 2011). Major sources of learning evolve from socializing experiences, social role models, collaboration with peers, and direct engagement with the beliefs, roles, and culture of the environment (Wilkerson & Irby, 1998). These experiences allow learning leaders to self-regulate, self-assess, self-reflect, and begin to develop perceptions about self-efficacy. Vygotsky describes a zone of proximal development (ZPD) as a social learning mechanism. The ZPD is a space where aspiring professionals observe and interact with more experienced practitioners to practice, receive feedback, and reflect on their performance (Papir-Bernstein, 2018; Vygotsky, 1978).

Ultimately, the success of our efforts to create knowledge-sharing collaborative cultures depends largely on our persuasive abilities to sell the idea of working together. Not everyone is open to this idea, but we can learn about theories of influence as in the fields of psychology and marketing to enhance our persuasive skills. Cialdini identified four key principles of social influence to consider when working with other professionals (Cialdini, 2001; Livingston, 2010; Papir-Bernstein, 2018): reciprocity, demonstrated by appreciating favors and exchanges; commitment and consistency through diligence; social proof from others who speak well of our efforts; and authority through administrative support.

It is not surprising that the concept of professional learning communities as collaborative work environments evolved from the world of business. In fact, PLCs reflect the evolving collaborative culture that is happening not only in business, but also in health care and education. This is a change from the recent history of most fields of practice, which was characterized by dominant paradigms of autonomy and isolation (Banks & Knuth, 2013; Papir-Bernstein, 2018). PLCs are based on the premise that reflections about daily experiences are enhanced when shared during interactions with other like-minded professionals.

Let's take a small sidestep and examine the shifting landscape of scientific stories that have influenced belief systems and perspectives about organizational cultures. Understanding this history helps us appreciate why it sometimes feels more difficult to work with and learn from each other than it does to work by ourselves. In her book, Lynne McTaggart (2008) explains that our stories define our lives, and help us make sense of all that goes on around us. It is our scientific stories, and specifically those about our universe, that most define us. We have grown up thinking that science presents the ultimate truth. Isaac Newton and Charles Darwin were both major authors of the story of our world. Both of their stories idealized separateness, competition, winning and losing, and that is how our world was fashioned. These stories formed the backbone of modern science, creating a worldview and overall frame for education and professional success: all elements of the universe are wholly self-contained and isolated from each other. Quantum physics and the quantum energy field tell a very different story. The quantum field binds us all together in a type of invisible web. At our universal essence, we exist in unity, in relationship, utterly interdependent with and affecting each part of the whole. Everything we do and think matters, because we are a part of something much larger. If we are not really separate there can be no winning and losing, and we would therefore have to redesign the choices we make governing our communities, our interactions and our work practices (Papir-Bernstein, 2018).

Although much of this research was conducted more than 30 years ago, it seems that our CoP are finally catching up. The concepts of knowledge-sharing and collaborative learning environments are certainly not new. They have been flagged in health care for over 40 years and advocated by the Institute of Medicine and more recently by the Institute for Healthcare Improvement, the World Health Organization, and the Interprofessional Education Collaborative. Within educational policy, the response to intervention (RTI) along with state education standards are driving the need for more extensive interprofessional collaborations (ASHA, 2016).

The American-Speech-Language-Hearing Association (ASHA) has long acknowledged the role of interprofessional education (IPE) and interprofessional practice (IPP) as critical for improving communication among professionals in health care and education. IPP occurs when multiple individuals from different professional backgrounds work together to provide comprehensive health care or educational services of the highest quality to individuals, their families, caregivers, and communities. A thoroughly informative publication grew out of an initiative by the ASHA Board of Special Interest Group Coordinators (BSIGC) to support an objective they titled Advance Interprofessional Education and Interprofessional Collaborative Practice (IPE/IPP), which was part of ASHA's 2015–2025 Strategic Pathway to Excellence (ASHA 2014b, 2015b, 2016). For a full discussion, webinars, convention resources, conference reports, and upcoming events about IPE and IPP, please see the ASHA IPP/IPE link.

Internal Communications

As stated earlier in the chapter, social supports linked to organizational communications act as a buffer to burnout. Asibey Consulting (2008) points out that the terms *communication* and *communications* are often used interchangeably, however, they have very different meanings. Communications refer to the channels and methods used for communication, such as person-to-person engagement, email, written reports, and websites. Along with organizational policies that facilitate the continuing goals and objectives of an organization so that it can accomplish its mission and vision, policies should also be established to facilitate communications objectives and priorities. One of these policies should require annual evaluation of the effectiveness of the organization's communications system and programs (Burrus & Willis, 2017). The goal of a communications evaluation should be "to establish whether or not the right information is getting to the right people, at the right time, by the right method, through the right channels" (National Association of Secondary School Principals [NASSP], 1990, p. 1).

Some common evaluation techniques include interviews, focus groups, surveys, observations, and quantitative data collection and analysis. Interviews are often conducted with a representative sample of individuals, and contain targeted yet open-ended questions that encourage divergent responses. Focus groups are effective for eliciting reactions to new policies, or group discussion about particular issues. Surveys can be done online or in person, and can contain a number of different formats. Appendix 8–B is an example of a survey used in a Department of Education speech therapy administrative unit. Observation is conducted to see how individuals or groups respond to specific communications. Quantitative data can be collected through surveys, social media networks, websites, or blogs. Results need to be analyzed, summarized and presented to interested parties. (Asibey, 2008; Krueger & Casey, 2000).

The major objective of a communications evaluation is to pinpoint specific communications strengths and weaknesses at an organization. For example, a survey can assess senders and receivers of information, the message content, the methods, the routes, the situations and the responses. Each of these key elements is affected by the organizational climate and interpersonal relationships. The following elements warrant evaluation (NASSP, 1990):

1. Communications ethics: This involves standards and practices implementing honesty, consistency, transparency, and protection of privacy. In order for communications to be considered ethical, information must be used for service to people rather than for positions of power.

2. Communications climate: Climate consists of general perceptions of an organization and its members. It includes the general mood or atmosphere at a particular time during communications or the context when the message is sent and received. Effective communications demand a healthy climate.

3. Communications channels (the "where"): Channels include the formal and informal routes or networks established for the reception and distribution of communications throughout the organization. Channels involve the direction of communications flow, such as upward, downward, and lateral, relative to chain of command. When considering flow, differences in rank, position, degree, age, and seniority are best minimized.

4. Communications methods (the "how"): Methods are divided into three categories: verbal, written, and digital. Each category can be formal or informal. Formal methods, such as memos or conferences, take planning and emphasize the needs of the organization. Informal methods, such as a casual conversation or a note, are usually unplanned and emphasize the needs of the sender.

5. Communications content (the "what"): The content is the substance of the communication, and can contain facts, ideas, and feelings.

6. Communications timing (the "when"): Appropriate timing is essential for messages to have maximum impact. Timing considers variables such as frequency, spacing, existing circumstances, and events occurring immediately before and after the message. Timing can be

affected by time of day, day of week, time of month, time of year, and the most receptive time for the receiver.

7. Communications sources (the "who"): All members of the organization are sources of information. Please verify if this is the intended meaning. Credible sources of information are candid, current, correct, clear, and relevant.

8. Communications feedback: Feedback, or the response, is a vital verification tool. Effective communications require feedback from the receiver, letting the sender know if the intent and content of the communications was understood.

Many of us spend much of our day communicating through meetings, emails, phone calls, generating reports, group discussion, and presentations or simply having conversations. We communicate constantly, so we need our communications to be effective. Mindtools (2017) has developed an easy to remember checklist of 7 Cs for effective internal communications:

- Be *clear*, by stating your purpose and communicating transparently.
- Be *concise*, by keeping it as brief as possible and sticking to your point.
- Be *concrete*, by using vivid images and laser-like focus.
- Be *correct*, by modeling technical and grammatical accuracy.
- Be *coherent*, by connecting all supporting points to the main message.
- Be *complete*, by supplying all necessary information so that your audience is informed and can take action.
- Be *courteous*, by facilitating an open, honest, and respectful process.

Internal communications can be one of the most difficult challenges leaders face, even for those in the communication industry. Communications are an implicit part of organizational effectiveness, and reflect culture, information flow, knowledge management, resource implementation, and strategy development. Internal communications influence key components of organizational success, such as employee retention, satisfaction, performance, and engagement. For reasons pertaining to professional expertise and ego, it may be difficult for leaders to admit that there are, in fact, communications dysfunctions in their organization. Matha and Boehm (2008) posit the need for *on-strategy* communications, a philosophy of communication that values simplicity and clarity and focuses organizations on understanding and delivering strategy when conducting their business. When organizational communications are on strategy, they focus the organization by clarifying direction, making communications relevant, preparing leadership to engage employees, and establishing ongoing conversations in all directions. The on strategy approach goes beyond what most people consider organizational communications, because it lives in the spaces between resources, management, leadership, and development. It becomes a driver for employee motivation, understanding, and execution.

Accountability and Verification

As leaders in our field, we know there are different levels of accountability, or practice verification. We are accountable to our coworkers, bosses, clients, and mostly to ourselves. Accountability is generally of two types. One level is local, or internal, and the other is global, or external (Stricker & Trierweiler, 2006). In the world of research, external verification happens through peer review and scientific discovery. In the world of practice, it happens through insurance agencies and other agencies that monitor our services. External verification is the major driver of reimbursement for health care and educational services and it usually requires documentation of some type. External documentation requirements change in health care and education as laws change, whereas organizational documentation requirements change as leadership changes.

Internal accountability is at least equally as important as external verification. Internal verification refers to the personal monitoring of professional practices and is client or organizationally based. One of the basic tenets of evidence-based practice (EBP) is that clinicians be sensitive and responsive to the specific needs, preferences, and values of clients and their caregivers (ASHA, 2005; Papir-Bernstein, 2018).

When people examine feelings about their own account-ability to a larger organization, they often view it strictly in terms of individual responsibility (Connors, Smith, & Hickman, 1994). As a result, responsibilities tend to fall through the cracks when they fall outside the boundaries drawn around independent aspects of an individuals' jobs. However, if accountability is viewed as something larger, people feel responsible for things beyond the literal interpretation of job descriptions. In other words, by adapting an attitude of "100-100" rather than "50-50," the cracks and boundaries disappear. What does the expression "50-50" refer to? It represents the idea that people are expected to share responsibility with others, half and half. However, we now know that the only formula that facilitates a win-win is 100-100 (Papir-Bernstein, 1995, 2018).

At the beginning of the chapter we talked about the meaning metric, and the importance of establishing ownership of it. As people establish ownership, they can better acknowledge their uniqueness, talents, tendencies, and fears. When they do not establish ownership, they become victims of circumstance, of personalities, and of bureaucracy. Conners, Smith, and Hickman (1994) discuss the concept of playing victim as it relates to accountability, saying that it holds people captive with little control over their circumstances. They blame others and point fingers. They focus more on what they cannot do rather than what they can do. The feel treated unfairly and powerless to change it. They get defensive, view the world with a pessimistic attitude, and say negative things about others.

The victim cycle runs through many phases, however six basic phases are common to most people and organizations (Papir-Bernstein, 2001, 2018):

1. Ignore or deny responsibility: a typical beginning point
2. "It's not my job": excuses inaction, redirects blame, and avoids responsibility
3. Finger pointing: denies responsibility for poor results and shifts blame to others
4. Confusion or "tell me what to do": relieves individuals of accountability; insisting on confusion makes it easier to do nothing about a situation
5. Cover your tail: crafting elaborate stories to avoid blame for something that goes wrong

6. Wait and see: choosing inactivity and hoping that things will improve without any action on an individual's part

The new accountability relates to ownership—rising above circumstances and doing whatever it takes to get the job done. It is about wondering, "What else can I do?," rather than thinking, "It's not my job." Accountability incorporates a perspective of balance and harmony, and embraces current and future efforts rather than reactive and historical excuses. A thin line separates feeling victimized from feeling accountable. As accountability deepens and professionals move above the line within the organization, a shift occurs from "Tell me what to do," to "Here is what I am going to do; what do you think?" Below are some suggestions for how professionals can move above the line (Conners et al.,1994; Papir-Bernstein, 2001, 2018)?

- Invite candid feedback about performance.
- Muster the courage to see reality, acknowledge problems, and welcome challenges.
- Don't waste time or energy on things you cannot control or influence.
- Commit 100% to what tasks and responsibilities, and if commitment begins to wane, rekindle it.
- Own the circumstances.
- Recognize when you are dropping below the line, and act quickly to avoid the traps of the victim cycle.
- Enjoy opportunities to make things happen.
- Constantly ask yourself "What more can I do to get the results I want?"

Summary

Leadership wellness begins with self-care and extends through organizational communications. This chapter explored topics related to personal attitudes, marketing and branding, advocacy, professional impairment and burnout, the impact of our work environment on stress and productivity, strategies for managing stress, the importance of creating knowledge-sharing cultures, professional accountability, and internal communications.

Experiential Commentary

Self-care needs to be addressed in professional life and in personal life. Many individuals are wonderful at care giving, and this was certainly true of me. It was not unusual take my work home, especially when I was involved with an organizational writing project. My home computer was actually gifted the title of "caregiver of the year," because it facilitated the birth of our organizational assessment and intervention guides. It is because I expected so much of myself that I also expected much of the people with whom I worked. I eventually learned to manage my time differently, minimize distractions, and accomplish more when in my office.

When I consider the impact of environmental stress factors, many examples come to mind. One has to do with the impact of clutter, which I had to squarely address, because it was having a profound impact on the appearance of one practitioner and the behaviors of the students in her speech therapy program. Materials and papers on the shelves in her therapy space lacked any sense of order or organization. Things were piled high and looked dangerously balanced. The room was sloppy, disorganized, and was an ongoing distractions for students. We came up with a plan to organizing and discard unneeded items, and during my next visit I saw significant changes. Students were better able to attend and communicate, and the practitioner presented a more professional appearance.

A second example of an environmental stress factor that I addressed in my supervisory programs is lighting. One practitioner under my supervision was exhibiting symptoms including unusual pallor, lack of motivation, and decreased affect in her communications. We spoke, and she was very honest about her feelings. I noticed that the lights in her therapy space were fluorescent, with one bulb out and the other one flickering. We talked about the importance of lighting, and whether she experienced these symptoms more in the winter than the summer. When she told me she did, I asked her to research Seasonal Affective Disorder (SAD), and that we would talk again soon. The next time I visited her, she had bought and was using a full spectrum lamp both at work and in her home. Her complete manner was back to where it had previously been. She told me that not only was she feeling better, but that she noticed a remarkable difference in the outcomes that some of her students were achieving.

Reflection

1. Describe your current physical, mental, social, emotional, environmental and spiritual strategies for self-care in your office. Are there any strategies you use successfully at home that you might be able to incorporate into your work setting?
2. Construct an elevator speech for the purpose of funding a particular initiative within your organization.
3. Familiarize yourself with ASHA's advocacy portal, and use all available resources to follow legislative issues discussed on the website. Take action by suggesting to staff members that they consider writing letters of support to their legislative representatives.
4. Think about coworkers who have exhibited signs of burnout or stress. What organizational variables may have contributed, and how have physical or social factors been ameliorated? If your organization does not have a wellness vision, how might you initiate one and what might be included?
5. What strategies are used in your organization for sharing knowledge? How is tacit experiential learning highlighted and validated?
6. Describe how your organization supports their implementation of professional learning communities through their use of social supports, collaborations, networks, and communities of practice.
7. If you were involved in evaluating organizational communications, how would you explain the need for that type of assessment, and how could you best implement the results of such a survey?
8. Explain two strategies for facilitating acknowledgment of organizational ownership among your coworkers.

References

Allen, J. (2008). *Wellness leadership: Creating supportive environments for healthier and more productive employees.* Retrieved from http://www.healthyculture.com

Allen, J., Hunnicutt, D., & Johnson, J. (1999). *Fostering wellness leadership: A new model.* Special Report from the Wellness Councils of America: Omaha, Nebraska.

American Speech-Language-Hearing Association. (n.d.-a). *Advocacy.* Available from http://www.asha.org/advocacy/

American Speech-Language-Hearing Association. (n.d.-b). *State advocacy.* Available from http://www.asha.org/advocacy/state/

American Speech-Language-Hearing Association. (2005). *Evidence-based practice in communication disorders* [Position statement]. Available from http://www.asha.org/policy

American Speech-Language-Hearing Association. (2014a). *Standards for the certificate of clinical competence in speech-language pathology.* Retrieved from http://www.asha.org/Certification/2014-Speech-Language-Pathology-Certification-Standards/

American Speech-Language-Hearing Association. (2014b). *Strategic pathway to excellence: 2015–2025.* Retrieved from http://www.asha.org/uploadedFiles/ASHA-Strategic-Pathway-to-Excellence.pdf

American Speech-Language-Hearing Association. (2015a). *Proposed revised standards for accreditation of graduate education programs in audiology and speech-language pathology.* Retrieved from http://caa.asha.org/wp-content/uploads/Accreditation-Standards-for-Graduate-Programs.pdf

American-Speech-Language-Hearing Association. (2015b). *Interprofessional education/interprofessional practice (IPE/IPP).* Rockville, MD: Author. Retrieved from http://www.asha.org/Practice/Interprofessional-Education-Practice/

American Speech-Language-Hearing Association. (2016). *Interprofessional education and interprofessional practice in communication sciences and disorders: An introduction and case-based examples of implementation in education and health care settings* [E-book]. Retrieved from http://www.asha.org/uploadedFiles/IPE-IPP-Reader-eBook.pdf

American Speech-Language-Hearing Association. (2017). Empowerment Zone. ASHA Convention. Los Angeles, CA. Available from http://www.asha.org/Events/convention/Empowerment-Zone/

American Speech-Language-Hearing Association Changing Healthcare Landscape Summit (ASHA CHLS). (2012). *Executive summary.*

Retrieved from https://www.asha.org/uploadedFiles/ASHA/Practice/Health-Care-Reform/Healthcare-Summit-Executive-Summary-2012.pdf

Asibey Consulting for the Communications Network. (2008). *Are we there yet? A communications evaluation guide.* Retrieved from https://www.luminafoundation.org/files/resources/arewethereyet.pdf

Banks, P., & Knuth, R. (2013). Working as a team: The new conception of professionalism. *ASHA SIG 16 Perspectives on School-Based Issues, 14,* 18–21.

Bradburn, N. (1969). *The structure of psychological well-being.* Chicago, IL: Aldine.

Burrus, A. E., & Willis, L. B. (2017). *Professional communication in speech-language pathology: How to write, talk, and act like a clinician.* San Diego, CA: Plural.

Cialdini, R. B. (2001). *Influence: Science and practice.* Boston, MA: Allyn & Bacon.

Clark, C. (2017). Seeking civility among faculty. *The ASHA Leader, 22,* 52–59.

Clark, M. K., & Flynn, P. (2011). Rational thinking in school-based practice. *Language, Speech and Hearing Services in Schools, 42,* 73–76.

Cobb, S. (1976). Social support as a moderator of life stress. *Psychosomatic Medicine, 5,* 300–317.

Conners, R., Smith, T., & Hickman, C. (1994). *The OZ principle: Getting results through individual and organizational accountability.* Upper Saddle River, NJ: Prentice Hall.

Ellis, K. C., Gottfred, C., & Freiberg, C. (2015). Minute to win it: Using elevator speeches to advocate in educational speech-language pathology and audiology. *Perspectives on School-Based Issues, 16,* 99–104.

Felt. A. (2014). Battling burnout: Change is possible with insight and effort. *Advance Newsmagazine.* King of Prussia, PA: Merion.

Flasher, L. V., & Fogle, P. T. (2012). *Counseling skills for speech-language pathologists and audiologists* (2nd ed.). Clifton Park, NY: Delmar Cengage Learning.

Fullan, M. G. (1990). *Changing school culture through staff development.* Alexandria, VA: Association for Supervision and Curriculum Development (ASCD).

Gardner, A. L., & Brindis, C. D. (2017). *Advocacy and policy change evaluation: Theory and practice.* Stanford, CA: Stanford University Press.

Gelles, D., & Miller, C. C. (2017, December 26). Schools teach M.B.A.s perils of "bro" ethos. *New York Times.* Retrieved from https://www.nytimes.com/2017/12/25/business/mba-business-school-ethics.html

Gupta, J. N. D., & Sharma, S. K. (2004). *Creating knowledge-based organizations.* Boston, MA: Idea Group.

Hafler, J. P. (2011). *Extraordinary learning in the workplace.* New York, NY: Springer.

Haidt, J. (2006). *The happiness hypothesis.* New York, NY: Basic Books

Hale, S. T., Kellum, G. D., & Burger, C., (2006, November). *Burnout in speech-language pathologists employed in schools.* Seminar presented at ASHA Convention, Miami Beach, FL.

Harris, I. B. (2011). Conceptions and theories of learning for workplace education. In J. P. Hafler (Ed.), *Extraordinary learning in the workplace.* (pp. 39–62). New York, NY: Springer.

Heaton, J. (2016). Tronvig group brand pyramid [Blog post]. Retrieved from http://www.tronviggroup.com/brand-pyramid/

Henri, B. P. (2011). At the table or on the table: It's our choice. *Perspectives on Administration and Supervision, 21*(1), 3–8.

Huffington, A. (2015). *Thrive: The third metric to redefining success and creating a life of well-being, wisdom, and wonder.* New York, NY: Harmony Books.

Human Resources Institute (HRI). (2011). *Wellness leadership: Part of the wellness culture coaching white paper series.* Retrieved from http://www.healthyculture.com/products_trainings.html

Innovation Network (IN). (2008). *Speaking for themselves: Advocates' perspectives on evaluation* [Research report]. Retrieved from http://www.innonet.org/client_docs/File/advocacy/speaking_for_them selves_web_enhanced.pdf

Kerka, S. (1995). The learning organization: Myths and realities. *Eric Clearinghouse on Adult, Career, and Vocational Education.* Retrieved from http://files.eric.ed.gov/fulltext/ED388802.pdf

Krueger, R. A., & Casey, M. A. (2000). *Focus groups: A practical guide for applied research.* Beverly Hills, CA: Sage.

Langdon, H., & Langdon Starr, M. (2014, November). *Resting is for more than just your voice: Self-care for SLPs.* Seminar presented at ASHA Convention, Orlando, FL.

LaRowe, K. (2008). *Breath of relief: Transforming compassion fatigue into flow.* Boston, MA: Acanthus.

Livingston, A. (2010). Supervision: Essentials of collaboration. *Perspectives on Administration and Supervision, 20,* 35–39.

Lubinski, R., & Hudson, M. (2013). *Professional issues in speech-language pathology and audiology.* New York, NY: Delmar Cengage Learning.

Maslow, A. H. (1968). *Toward a psychology of being.* New York, NY: D. Van Nostrand.

Matha, B., & Boehm, M. (2008). *Beyond the babble: Leader communication that drives results*. Hoboken, NJ: Wiley.

McTaggart, L. (2008). *The field*. New York, NY: HarperCollins.

Michael J. Fox Foundation (MJFF). (2014). *Clinical trials recruitment best practices manual (PDF)*. For researchers: Trial resources. Retrieved from https://www.michaeljfox.org/files/MJFF_Recruitment_Best_Practices_manual.pdf

Mindtools. (2017). *The 7 Cs of communication: A checklist for clear communication* [Online article]. Retrieved from https://www.mind tools.com/pages/article/newCS_85.htm

National Association of Secondary School Principals (NASSP): The Practitioner. (1990). *Assessing the communications effectiveness of your school*, (17), (2), 1–12.

Nonaka, I. (1994). A dynamic theory of organizational knowledge creation. *Organizational Science, 5*(1), 14–37.

Nonaka, I., & Hirotaka, T. (1995). *The knowledge creating company: How Japanese companies create the dynamics of innovation*. Oxford, UK: Oxford University Press.

O'Dell, C., & Grayson, C. J. (1998). *If only we knew what we know: The transfer of internal knowledge and best practice*. New York, NY: The Free Press

Papir-Bernstein, W. (1995). *Supervision for the 21st century: Facilitating self-directed professional growth*. Seminar presented at the New York State Speech-Language-Hearing Association (NYSSLHA), New York, NY.

Papir-Bernstein, W. (2001, November). *Creating the perfect fit: Merging personal competence with program effectiveness*. Seminar presented at ASHA Convention, New Orleans, LA.

Papir-Bernstein, W. (2012a). The artistry of practice-based evidence (PBE): One practitioner's path—Part I. In R. Goldfarb (Ed.), *Translational speech-language pathology and audiology* (pp. 51–57). San Diego, CA: Plural.

Papir-Bernstein, W. (2012b). The artistry of practice-based evidence (PBE): One practitioner's path—Part II. In R. Goldfarb (Ed.), *Translational speech-language pathology and audiology* (pp. 83–89). San Diego, CA: Plural.

Papir-Bernstein, W. (2018). *The practitioner's path in speech-language pathology: The art of school-based practice*. San Diego, CA: Plural.

Papir-Bernstein, W., & Legrand, R. (1993). *Differentiated systems for staff development: Self direction and reflection*. Seminar presented at ASHA Convention, Anaheim, CA.

Pfifferling, J. (1986). Cultural antecedents promoting professional impairment. In C. D. Scott & J. Hawk (Eds.), *Heal thyself: The health of health care professionals.* (pp. 3–18). New York, NY: Brunner/ Mazel.

Pickering, J., & Embry, E. (2013). So long, silos. *The ASHA Leader, 18,* 38–45.

Pines, A. (1982). Changing organizations: Is a work environment without burnout a possible goal? In W. S. Paine (Ed.), *Job stress and burnout.* Beverly Hills, CA: Sage.

Pines, A. (1986). Who is to blame for helpers' burnout? Environmental impact. In C. D. Scott & J. Hawk (Eds.), *Heal thyself: The health of health care professionals.* (pp. 19–43). New York, NY: Brunner/Mazel.

Pines, A., & Aronson, E. (1988). *Career burnout: Causes and cures.* New York, NY: Free Press.

Polovoy, C. (2015). What are you selling? *The ASHA Leader, 20*(12), 34–35. doi:10.1044/leader.IPP.20122015.34

Redding, W. C. (1972). *Communication within the organization.* New York, NY: Industrial Communication Council.

Ross, E. (2011). Burnout and self-care in the professions of speech pathology and audiology: An ecological perspective. In R. J. Fourie (Ed.), *Therapeutic processes for communication disorders: A guide for clinicians and students.* (pp. 213–228). New York, NY: Psychology Press.

Rudebusch, J., & Wiechmann, J. (2013). The SLP's guide to PLCs. *Perspectives on School-Based Issues, 14,* 22–27.

Ruder, K., Noplock, M. L., & Johnson, P. R. (2003). Grassroots legislative advocacy. *Perspectives on Administration and Supervision, 13*(2), 46.

Schaufeli, W. B., Leiter, M. P., & Maslach, C. (2009). Burnout: 35 years of research and practice. *Career Development International, 14*(3), 204–220.

Scott, C. D., & Hawk, J. (Eds.). (1986). *Heal thyself: The health of health care professionals.* New York, NY: Brunner/Mazel.

Scott, C. R. (2007). Communication and social identity theory: Existing and potential linkages in organizational identification research. *Communication Studies, 58,* 123–138.

Seligman, M. E. P. (2011). *Flourish: A new understanding of happiness and well-being—and how to achieve them.* London, UK: Nicholas Brealey.

Senge, P. (2006). *The fifth discipline: The art and practice of the learning organization.* New York, NY: Doubleday.

Silver, N. (2012). *The signal and the noise: Why so many predictions fail —but some don't.* New York, NY: The Penguin Press.

Singletary, F. F., & Smith, M. P. (2014, November). *Using a research registry to recruit for clinical trials.* Poster presented at ASHA Convention, Orlando, FL.

Sjodin, T. (2012*). Small message, big impact: The elevator speech effect.* New York, NY: Penguin Group.

Skinner, S. (2001). *Feng shui: Before and after.* Boston, MA: Tuttle.

Smith, B. H. (1981). Narrative versions, narrative theories. In W. J. T. Mitchell (Ed.), *On narrative.* (pp. 209–232). Chicago, IL: University of Chicago Press.

Smith, M. K. (2001). The learning organization: Principles, theory and practice. *Infed.org.* Retrieved from http://www.infed.org/biblio/learning-organization.htm

Stricker, G., & Trierweiler, S. J. (2006). The local scientist: A bridge between science and practice. *Training and Education in Professional Psychology,* S(1),37–46.

Sue, V. M., & Ritter, L. A. (2007). *Using online surveys in evaluation.* San Francisco, CA: Jossey-Bass.

Texas Medical Association. (2010). *Three stages of burnout.* Retrieved from http://smhp.psych.ucla.edu/qf/burnout_qt/3stages.pdf

Vygotsky, L. S. (1978). Interaction between learning and development. In C. Michael (Ed.), *Mind in society: The development of higher psychological processes* (pp. 79–91). Cambridge, MA: Harvard University Press.

Wilkerson, L., & Irby, D. (1998). Strategies for improving teaching practice: A comprehensive approach to faculty development. *Academic Medicine, 73,* 387–396.

World Health Organization. (1997). *WHOQOL: Measuring quality of life.* Geneva, Switzerland: Author.

Wright, P., & Wright, P. (2016). *From emotions to advocacy: The special education survival guide.* Deltaville, VA: Harbor House Law Press.

APPENDIX 8–A
Leadership Wellness Support

Wendy Papir-Bernstein (Adapted from HRI, 2011)

The following survey assesses the quality and quantity of leadership support for organizational wellness. Please rate your level of agreement with the following statements using the following scale:

1 Strongly disagree, 2 Disagree,
3 Neither agree nor disagree, 4 Agree, 5 Strongly agree

The organizational leader:

1. Explains why wellness is important to the organization.

    1   2   3   4   5

2. Explains how employees can benefit from wellness.

    1   2   3   4   5

3. Explains how employees can participate in a wellness program.

    1   2   3   4   5

4. Demonstrates support for wellness through personal choices.

    1   2   3   4   5

5. Participates in wellness by modeling wellness activities.

    1   2   3   4   5

6. Adopts stress management policies and procedures.

    1   2   3   4   5

7. Participates in setting organizational wellness goals.

    1   2   3   4   5

8. Reduces barriers to achieving wellness goals.

1   2   3   4   5

9. Celebrates individual and shared wellness achievements

1   2   3   4   5

Reference

Human Resources Institute (HRI). (2011). *Wellness leadership: Part of the wellness culture coaching white paper series.* Retrieved from http://www.healthyculture.com/Articles/Wellness%20Leadership%20White%20Paper.pdf

APPENDIX 8-B

Communications Effectiveness Survey

Wendy Papir-Bernstein (Adapted from NASSP, 1990)

The following survey assesses the components of communication effectiveness. Please rate your level of agreement with the following statements using the following scale:

1 Strongly disagree, **2** Disagree,
3 Neither agree nor disagree, **4** Agree, **5** Strongly agree

I. Communications Ethics

1. Confidential information is identified and protected.

       1   2   3   4   5

2. Staff member's rights to privacy are respected and safeguarded.

       1   2   3   4   5

3. Information is provided internally before released to the public.

       1   2   3   4   5

4. Management's actions are consistent with its words.

       1   2   3   4   5

5. All people are informed of expectations, rights, and responsibilities.

       1   2   3   4   5

6. People are supplied with information necessary to do their jobs.

       1   2   3   4   5

7. Reasons for important decisions and actions are shared with honesty.

1   2   3   4   5

II. Communications Climate

1. People are approachable and available to each other.

1   2   3   4   5

2. Status and position are less important than how people are treated.

1   2   3   4   5

3. Management projects an attitude of care and value.

1   2   3   4   5

4. People feel respected, listened to, and responded to.

1   2   3   4   5

5. A feeling of mutual trust exists between fellow workers.

1   2   3   4   5

6. Sensitive problems and serious conflicts are faced and discussed candidly.

1   2   3   4   5

7. Leadership is receptive to suggestions, and then follows up.

1   2   3   4   5

III. Communications Channels

1. Responsibility is fixed for organizing and coordinating important messages.

1   2   3   4   5

2. Approved channels for communications are identified and understood.

1   2   3   4   5

3. Horizontal or lateral communications exist among coworkers.

1   2   3   4   5

4. Upward vertical communication is comfortable and accessible.

1   2   3   4   5

5. Downward vertical communication is respectful and effective.

1   2   3   4   5

IV. Communications Methods

1. A wide variety of communications methods are used to convey information.

1   2   3   4   5

2. The method used is tailored to the content and receiver of the message.

1   2   3   4   5

3. Important information is presented verbally and in writing.

1   2   3   4   5

4. Opportunities for meaningful face-to-face discussion exist.

1   2   3   4   5

V. Communications Content

1. Message content is consistently factual and accurate.

1   2   3   4   5

2. Messages are carefully written and contain a logical sequence of ideas.

1   2   3   4   5

3. Wording of messages is adapted to the receiver and situation.

1   2   3   4   5

4. A variety of appropriate verbal, written, and digital channels are utilized.

1   2   3   4   5

5. Message content is important and relevant.

1   2   3   4   5

6. Messages sound credible, sincere, and to the point.

1   2   3   4   5

7. Message meanings are clear and require little or no interpretation by receivers.

1   2   3   4   5

VI. Communications Timing

1. Timing of important messages is carefully planned and coordinated.

1   2   3   4   5

2. Necessary information reaches people at opportune times.

1   2   3   4   5

3. People's questions and requests are responded to promptly.

1   2   3   4   5

4. Information about activities and deadlines is given with sufficient notice.

1   2   3   4   5

5. Important communications are appropriately spaced out.

    1   2   3   4   5

6. Urgent information reaches people promptly.

    1   2   3   4   5

VII. Communications Sources

1. All important information is written down and readily accessible.

    1   2   3   4   5

2. Sources of important information are trusted, credible, and knowledgeable.

    1   2   3   4   5

3. The people with information are viewed as cooperative and helpful.

    1   2   3   4   5

4. The policy manual is available, accurate, and up to date.

    1   2   3   4   5

5. Adequate opportunity exists for exchange of information with coworkers.

    1   2   3   4   5

6. Research is used as needed and results are shared.

    1   2   3   4   5

7. A communications plan exists for emergency information.

    1   2   3   4   5

VIII. Communications Feedback

1. A system exists for verifying that information was received and understood.

1   2   3   4   5

2. Provision is made to evaluate new practices following implementation.

1   2   3   4   5

3. The giving of feedback is a valued component of the organization.

1   2   3   4   5

4. Evaluation of the communications system occurs at least once a year.

1   2   3   4   5

Reference

National Association of Secondary School Principals (NASSP): The practitioner. (1990). *Assessing the communications effectiveness of your school*, XVII(2), 1–12.

9

Leadership Trends: What Is Trending in Leadership Practices?

Wendy Papir-Bernstein

Leadership is about making others better as a result of your presence, and making sure that impact lasts in your absence.

—Sheryl Sandberg

Learning Objectives

- The reader will learn about leadership universality and the trends that impact leadership in most fields today.
- The reader will learn how leadership innovations have and must continue to respond to changes in the clinical landscape.
- The reader will learn how to apply the concepts of boundary-spanning leadership, 360-degree leadership, and mindfulness to their own leadership practices.
- The reader will reflect upon the importance of expanding leadership cultivation within diverse and inclusive communities of practice.

Introduction

Whereas natural sciences (the physical universe and its laws) deal with the behavior of matter and energy, social sciences deal with the behavior of people and human institutions. The reality of natural sciences rarely changes, or if it does, it changes only after an earth shattering scientific discovery. On the other hand, the reality of social sciences is subject to constant change, and this means that assumptions we made yesterday can sometimes become outdated. In Peter Drucker's book about management trends (Drucker, 1999), he talks about assumptions humans make and how they drive trends. The paradigms, or prevailing theories, of all social sciences are based on assumptions we make about the reality we perceive. These assumptions are present in most professional disciplines, often determining what is attended to and ignored by scholars, writers, and practitioners. "Yet, despite their importance, the assumptions are rarely analyzed, rarely studied, rarely challenged—indeed rarely even made explicit" (Drucker, 1999, p. 3). As we change our assumptions, one might say that we are trendsetting.

Trends are very much a sign of the times, and relate to the zeitgeist of a particular era. *Zeitgeist* is a word of German derivation that roughly means "the spirit of an age, sensibility of an era, and the intellectual inclinations and biases that underlie human endeavor" as flavored by a particular period of history (Papir-Bernstein, 2018, p. 55). As a result of the zeitgeist, parallel trends appear in most creative enterprises, such as literature, architecture, and art, and extend to science, religion, health care, and education (Hendrix, 2005). In other words, once a trend catches, it becomes universal.

Another way of describing trends is through an understanding of the concept of fractals. A *fractal* is a never-ending pattern, a system of repetitions that run across dimensions. The concept evolved in mathematics and extended to nature and art. Fractals show up everywhere around us in all sciences. For example, the same geometry that describes the shape of coastlines explains the patterns of galaxies, the shape of a conch shell, and how stock prices soar and plummet. The viewing of fractals tend to be soothing because they are somewhat predictable, much like the routines we like to use when working with our clients (Edgar, 2004).

Many books that deal with trendsetting do so through a particular lens, such as business or industry, when in fact the challenges with which we are faced present themselves in almost all organizations of today's society. They impact education, health care, government, and industry—and usually for the same reasons. Methods must keep pace with changing societal trends and demands. Research in the area of cognitive science might explain it this way: when we make improvements to our leadership approaches, unfortunately they are often in the realm of single loop rather than double loop learning. *Single loop learning* (SLL) usually involves simple adjustments we make to existing techniques, and *double loop learning* (DLL) involves changes to our assumptions, perspectives, and frameworks on which our techniques and programs are based. Only with DLL is there potential for real change, because through reflective practices we can better align ideas with actions, and actions with outcomes (Argyis & Schon, 1996; Papir-Bernstein, 2012b; Petrie, 2014).

Any type of change, including trendsetting, brings with it strategic considerations impacted by social, economic, and policy factors. Leaders are stakeholders in the future of changemaking, and changemakers need to ask themselves the following questions (KnowledgeWorks, 2018):

- What is my motivation and vision for leadership?
- What scope of organizational change will best support changes in the broader landscape?
- How might decision-making authority need to shift?
- What new structures would best enable collaboration and coordination?

Tracking the Trends

The future cannot be created alone. Marketing expert and trend forecaster Faith Popcorn developed unique techniques for tracking trends, which are still used throughout diverse professions in our society. She would gather people together (who would not ordinarily work in the same space or even in the same profession), and encourage them to exchange ideas about a particular topic or problem. For example, she might call together a doctor, an architect, and a film director to discuss recycling. She called it her TalentBank (Popcorn, 1991). She explains that the future " . . . evolves from a confluence of psycho-social-demographic-economic factors" (p. 13). When you bring experts together from different disciplines to solve a problem, each expert glimpses a different part of the puzzle. As the pieces all come together to make a whole, the future takes form. She called it *brailling*, reaching out to touch as many parts of our culture as possible so that we develop a new sensitivity for what is really in front of us. Anticipating a new reality is the beginning of the creation process, and trend tracking helps us anticipate.

Trends present a map to the future and provide insight about feelings, moods, impulses, and motivations. The relationship between trends and impulses is one of the reasons trends have been termed *mood marketing*. Trends often start small and pick up momentum. If you suspect the coming of a possible trend, and then connect the dots between the inception of a trend and its impact on a profession, you can fine-tune your organization to ride or even embrace the wave (Popcorn, 1991). As you shape your organizational strategies around emerging trends, you will be *trendBending*, as Popcorn calls it (Popcorn, 1991). One way Popcorn suggests to get on trend is to imagine a language with only a future tense. She calls that *trendTalk*. When we *trendBend*, we discover what the trends have in common with the intrinsic qualities of our product and service, which impacts our vision and organizational objectives. Sometimes, in order to trendBend, we need to twist the familiar by changing something comfortable into something new.

Another of Popcorn's techniques is called *universal screening*, which is simply filtering whatever you look at or listen to through a *trend lens*. Most of us are confronted with so much visual and auditory information that we tend to screen out most of it subconsciously. Or, we pay attention to things we think apply to our lives as they exist in the present. The bottom line is that we tend to pay attention to the familiar; that is, to things we already recognize and know. By using the universal screen to sort input, we " . . . begin to recognize ways in which information that seems to have nothing to do with you might, in fact, have everything to do with you—and your business" (Popcorn, 1991, p. 115). As you apply your universal screen, you develop an instinctive, shorthand method of organizing what you need to know about the world's direction. You channel information for the future, and that is trendsetting.

As with any new concept or trend, there is usually a series of pendulum swings as we are cautioned against discarding the old for the new. Trends sometimes incorporate a new lens rather than new information; however, in either case, leaders must incorporate wisdom with perspective about integrating and culling rather, than simply discarding. That is the greatest challenge—keeping what works and changing what does not.

A New Leadership Universality

What are the truths and trends about the future that drive leadership in most industries? Ian Ziskin, president of a human capital coaching and consulting firm, describes leaders as visionaries who live at the intersection of preparation and opportunity (2015). He sees the emergence of a new and universal leadership title, that of *COCO: chief organizational capability officer*. The COCO recognizes and integrates innovation, talent, and opportunity for transformation within the existing organizational community. The power of leadership rests with creating the glue of leadership currency, connecting the dots and turbocharging the in-between points. Our professional glue facilitates the ability to look for, receive, and translate new concepts into meaningful directions for our work. It helps us understand that information is all around us, and comes to us sometimes from unexpected sources, crossing over from one field to another (Papir-Bernstein, 2012a).

COCOs appreciate that the leadership currency of choice often appears outside of the immediate environment, and has the ability to see around corners and through a variety of lenses and perspectives. So many of the challenges we now face are cross-functional and interdisciplinary in nature, and thus require collaborative and broad-based solutions that stretch us and extend our reach past traditional boundaries of time and space (Finney, 2013; Ziskin, 2016).

Another universal model of leadership presented by Bradberry and Greaves (2012) introduces the idea that leadership has both core and adaptive components. The core components are what influence some people to be perceived as born leaders. Core components include the implementation of strategies, which require vision, judgment, and planning; actions, which require decision-making and communication; and results, which require agility and focus.

On the other hand, adaptive components are practical, repeatable qualities that can be learned with a bit of effort. Adaptive leadership components involve emotional intelligence, organizational justice, character, and development. Emotional intelligence requires self-awareness, self-management, social awareness, and relationship management. Organizational justice requires fairness in decision-making, information-sharing, and concern about organizational outcomes. Character requires credibility and integrity, and development requires motivation for lifelong learning and investment in training others.

There is one additional leadership universality, which relates to generational shifts, and can be termed *generation-speak*. It seems to be driven by the generational influx of millennials and involves creating balance between individuals' personal and professional lives, as well as balance between performance and purpose. This trend in leadership practices has evolved to more of a holistic or whole person approach for well-rounded leaders (Ziskin, 2011). The need for balance compels us to approach our work with an understanding of our purpose, and a sense of appreciation that through our work we are fulfilling that purpose. Today, we ask questions: Why am I doing this work? How do I infuse my best work into the best aspects of society? How can I satisfy my sense of universal responsibility through my perspective as a professional and as an individual? Leaders today understand that while research provides information, it does not provide all we need to know. We model a harmonious interplay between qualitative practices and quantitative numbers, theory and practice, personal reflections and data, and science with inner ways of knowing (Papir-Bernstein, 2018).

Now is the time for some generation-speak (which might be construed as politically incorrect because it is not person first, so please forgive me). In a recent issue of *The ASHA Leader* (2017c), generations were a topic of discussion. In a generational survey, gathered as a component of ASHA membership data at the end of each year, Generation X represents the largest share of ASHA members (42%). As baby boomers (29% of ASHA members) retire, the millennials are coming up fast behind (27%; ASHA, 2017). What the survey could not address were the vast numbers of Generation Z, born after 1996 and largely the children of millennials, rising up through undergraduate and graduate programs. Defining characteristics of Generation Z include attention to visuals, love of challenges, desire for interaction, engagement, and immediate bottom lines (Combi, 2015). Professors and workforce leaders in the field, must tailor experiences to match learning and motivational styles of each generation of workers. (Roseberry-McKibbin, 2017).

A third leadership universality is the attention we pay to memes and memetic theory. Leaders inspire ideas to be developed and shared with others, and nurture them to grow and live on in the world. Why do some messages have lasting impact on opinions and behaviors? The study of memes, or *memetics*, seeks to answer that question. Memes consist of text over an image, short videos, or digital clip art meant to spread and be imitated. In the field of speech-language pathology, Kamhi (2004) first brought memetic theory to our attention when discussing titles SLPs choose to call themselves by professionally. In fact, the appeal of ideas lies neither with truth nor logic, but with a theory that originates from the field of evolution. A meme is actually a unit of imitation that helps explain why tunes and fashion fads are memorable, and why catch phrases are catchy (Altran, 2001; Papir-Bernstein, 2018). The study and proliferation of speech pathology memes is apparent on social networking sites, such as Instagram and Facebook.

Memes churn through culture at a blinding rate, and therefore sometimes provide shortcut marketing tools. Leaders need to be aware that they do exist and how they impact and shape the worldview of professionals and consumers. Why do some ideas (memes) catch on or "stick" and others do not? Heath and

Heath (2007) investigated the *stickiness factors*, and their implementation in social sciences, education, and medicine when one is conducting, disseminating, and applying research (Cook, Cook, & Landrum, 2013). Ideas with a strong stickiness factor tend to be (Papir-Bernstein, 2018):

- Simple: Strip an idea to its core and craft it so it resonates with the audience.
- Unexpected: Use elements of surprise to increase focus and generate interest.
- Concrete: Explain ideas in a way that relates to meaningful and functional human activities.
- Credible: Let them flow from personal and experiential stories, rather than data.
- Emotional: Connect the audience to people rather than to concepts.
- Storified: Use stories (an essential component of science) to effectively disseminate research findings.

Leadership Innovations Respond to Changes in the Clinical Landscape

Leadership innovations must meet the accelerating pace and complexity of challenges facing future leaders in every field and profession. The online resource known as The Center for Creative Leadership has identified variables that influence the need for leadership training in the business world: information overload, digital connectedness, dissolution of traditional organizational boundaries, generational differences and the accompanying diversity of values and expectations, and increased globalization (Kegan & Lahey, 2009; Roger & Petrie, 2017).

In the CSD field, we may refer to those variables with different terms, but the challenges are the same. In 2009 as an ASHA Advisory Councilor for New York, I met as a member of ASHA's Advisory Councils in Audiology and Speech-Language Pathology to study a document regarding societal trends, published by the American Society of Association Executives (2008). We, along with

ASHA's Board of Directors, ranked 50 external trends and sorted them into sociodemographic, economic, technological, political, and environmental categories that we felt could affect the future of CSD professions. Numerous themes emerged, including the societal impacts of generational differences, diversity, clinical populations, and technological (Lemke & Dublinski, 2010, 2011). These same trends still impact ASHA's vision, mission, core values, strategic themes, and objectives (ASHA, 2017a), and will certainly impact leadership development in the field. Each theme was analyzed for potential impact on the profession, and here are some of the conclusions drawn (Lemke & Dublinski, 2010).

Generational trends related to baby boomers will increase the number of retirements, resulting in staff shortages, and retraining/retooling needs of older staff members who decide to continue working. Generational trends related to millennials will increase the need for digital connectedness, opportunities for engagement and social activities, and staff development to addresses conflict resolution and negative work attitudes, and to encourage of innovation.

Diversity trends will continue to impact the need for diversity competence in practice and training programs to raise awareness of potential biases in all areas of diversity (e.g., age, socioeconomic status, disability, culture, sexual orientation, and gender identity).

Clinical population trends relate largely to the world's aging population and has implications for the design of products, services, and tools, as well as interdisciplinary training. This trend also impacts legislative policies, funding streams, health care budgets, reimbursement policies, the need for prevention awareness, wellness training, and overall health literacy.

Technology trends relate to practice tools, online education, social networking platforms, the possibility of telepractice for training programs and remote work settings, and changes in staff conferencing and communication formats.

In ongoing reports about changing *trends in the educational and health care landscapes*, ASHA discussed the need to reframe the perception of our professions (ASHA, 2013). ASHA stressed that leaders must stay informed about how changing trends impact the big picture of our clinical framework with regard to professional practice, research and data needs, professional preparation, interprofessional education (IPE), and interprofessional practice (IPP). The trends affect both the health care arena and educational settings. The goal is to increase value to individuals by delivering services that improve functional outcomes that matter to their everyday lives. Strategies were discussed, later implemented, and continue to be relevant to the current trends in the CSD field:

1. Develop functional goals, using the International Classification of Disabilities and Function (ICF) framework;
2. Enhance clinical outcome measures, using ASHA's National Outcomes Measurement System (NOMS) to document therapy;
3. Develop clinical practice portals to standardize clinical practice guidelines for specific diagnoses, conditions, and ages;
4. Implement telepractice and other technological advances to facilitate access for services;
5. Increase public awareness of how we participate in health literacy and communication wellness;
6. Develop roles for self-management at home, which may include employment of support personnel and training for patients and caregivers.

Value in health care is measured by outputs, or actual patient health outcomes. It is no longer measured by inputs, or volume of services delivered. More care is not always seen as better care; the focus has shifted from quantity to quality, from volume to value (Porter, 2010). In CSD, value is defined by client outcomes, rather than practitioner effort. We can only deliver value if we embrace strategic agility, balance a culture of accountability with a culture of creativity, and replace metrics with patient-centered functional outcomes (Rao, 2014). Value-based service is not really about reimbursement, although they may get tied together in the future.

McNeilly (2018) reminds us that we need to maximize time spent delivering the services that we are uniquely qualified to provide, and in that manner demonstrate our true value. It is critical that we continue to provide a range of service in a variety of settings to demonstrate that we do, in fact, practice at the top of our license. Thus, we must provide professional development on emerging practice strategies and work with clients and their families on self-management. Self-management empowers individuals to improve their level of functioning based on strategies designed but not implemented by an SLP. It may also help develop our own ability to delegate certain responsibilities to others, and engage in only those activities that require our level of expertise and skill.

Ongoing changes in outcome reporting, payment models, and reimbursement programs promote increased accountability and cost-effectiveness. Current trends drive the use of diverse service delivery options, such as telepractice and using assistants to deliver certain types of services. This allows us to provide the service we are uniquely qualified to provide and collaborate with service extenders to deliver the rest. As a result, we can delegate responsibilities that do not require professional interpretation and judgment, enhance our supervision and management skills, and contribute to team-building and communities of care. *Service extenders* include assistants, rehabilitation technicians, family members, and community workers. These service delivery options enhance value and functional outcomes for clients, and facilitate focusing on services that require our specialized training (ASHA, 2013; McNeilly, 2018).

Top of the practice becomes especially important because ASHA (2017b) reports that job opportunities for speech-language pathologists are expected to grow by 21% in the ten-year period that began in 2014, a larger average growth rate than in most other professions in the United States. There are many reasons for that growth, including the following:

1. Older populations are prone to medical conditions that can result in speech, language, and swallowing problems.
2. Current practitioners will retire from the field.
3. Medical advances will improve survival rate for infants born prematurely, stroke survivors, and trauma victims.
4. Young children with speech, language, and swallowing disorders will be identified earlier.
5. School enrollments will increase for children in regular and special education classes.

Knowledge Management

One of the main objectives of leadership in any organization is to improve performance outcomes. Organizational theorists suggest that organizational knowledge, in academia as well as business, is one of the most valuable commodities and strategic assets in an organization. For the last 25 years, many leaders have incorporated principles of knowledge management (KM) into their organizational mission and objectives. KM involves a systematic process of identifying, capturing, and transferring knowledge to the people in the organization who need it most. Leaders who use knowledge management are able to make better decisions faster, take action more consistent with needs, improve motivation, and energize innovation. However, internal structures are often so complex that knowledge sources are difficult to find, fragmented, inconsistent, contradictory, or under-utilized. (Leal & Roldan, 2001; Papir-Bernstein, 2012a; Tohidi & Jabbari, 2012).

We have become more adept at googling information in lieu of looking for and finding it within our own organizations. Organizational learning capacity is the ability of an organization to learn from experiences and pass them on through time and space. The distinction between horizontal and vertical development parallels the distinction between explicit and tacit knowledge. As the previous chapter discussed in detail, explicit knowledge, usually formal and more easily codified, comes from books, papers, and policy manuals. Tacit knowledge, on the other hand, is gained through experiences, perceptions, insights, and know-how—best communicated by people through shared experiences (Hildreth & Kimble, 2002; Papir-Bernstein, 2018). Tohidi and Jabbari report that close to 90% of the knowledge in any organization is embedded within the minds of individual workers, and has not been recorded into official training or professional development documents (2012). It remains invisible, and is often lost to the organization unless leadership makes better use of KM, which remains a largely under-tapped resource.

Knowledge gets transformed and utilized most efficiently when people trust and cooperate with each other. Knowledge assets must be recognized, acknowledged, and rewarded when shared. Comfortable and safe environments make that possible.

Whereas technology helps with the collection and codification of explicit knowledge for distribution, it does not get tacit knowledge out of someone's head. Only people can do that. Tacit knowledge and the establishment of modalities for sharing it, play key roles in the overall quality of knowledge application within an organization (Papir-Bernstein, 2018; Smith, 2001).

Leal and Roldan (2001), and more recently, Tohidi and Jabbari (2012) conducted research reviews of barriers to effective KM. Their findings suggest that the barriers can be divided into two main groupings: barriers to the creation of new knowledge, and barriers to knowledge transfer. Barriers to the creation of new knowledge include diversity of beliefs and cognitive abilities, lack of acknowledgment and incentives, and inertia and resistance to change. Barriers to knowledge transfer include lack of commitment, organizational mistrust, poor training, social isolation, and space restrictions.

As leaders, how do we create value in the transfer of knowledge and the sharing of tacit resources? We do it through benchmarking. Benchmark, used as a verb, means " . . . to systematically identify and learn from best practices, internal or external, in order to improve your own performance" (O'Dell & Grayson, 1998, p. xiv). Within a KM system, benchmarking facilitates individual and organizational learning. The idea that organizations need to be in a continuous learning mode is far from a new one. What is new, in the field of leadership, is to have tools in place that allow you to know what you are doing well to facilitate professional growth, and where new growth is necessary. The fine details of learning-focused leadership need to be described in ways that support and inform the practice of our craft. When we are able to do that, we will enhance our organization, support our discipline, and prepare for its future.

Boundary-Spanning Leadership

In order for organizations to truly be innovative, they must develop leaders throughout their structure. In fact, the organization of the future is one where everyone is a leader because they are empowered to lead themselves. Leadership must be developed within every individual working in the organization. As leaders who need to create direction, alignment, and commitment to working across boundaries, we need to work across differences that traditionally divide us. Spanning boundaries creates opportunities for broadened perspectives, client partnerships, employee empowerment at all levels, expanded collaborations, new learning, and organizational innovations. Some of the societal trends that speak to the importance of boundary-spanning leadership are diversity and generational differences, global mindsets, and technological advances (Charan, Drotter, & Noel, 2000; Ernst & Chrobot-Mason, 2010).

Maxwell (2011) describes two organizational strategies from the Center for Creative Leadership to build boundary-spanning capabilities that focused on developing leadership talent and leadership culture. Talent development involves an organization's ability to attract, prepare, and retain professionals with the capabilities to facilitate organizational success. Culture development requires understanding the individual and collective beliefs and practices that produce organizational outcomes (Yip, Ernst, & Campbell, 2016).

Effective leaders bring value and influence to every level of an organization by becoming 360-degree leaders. That means they can learn to lead up, lead down, and lead across, as they exert influence in all directions and span vertical and horizontal boundaries. Vertical boundaries move across levels and established hierarchies. Horizontal boundaries move across functions and expertise. Leading up involves a leader's administrators, superiors, and bosses. It requires understanding of your boss's communication preferences (how much and how often). Leading down involves a leader's subordinates (the people they manage). It requires strong mentoring and coaching skills as well as an understanding of generational and cultural differences. Leading across involves members of your own team (your peers; Maxwell, 2011). The trick is to develop the ability to influence people all around you in your organization, and to be able to do it from any vantage point (Yip, Ernst, & Campbell, 2016).

We sometimes have a tendency to wait for the title and the position before exerting our influence. Authority is not necessarily given, but it is always assumed. Maxwell (2011) describes the authority aspect of leadership as existing on a staircase. The following five steps are dynamic, and where each leader stands varies with their history. The authority of most leaders begins with the first step but they do not always move up the staircase. The good news is that leaders can increase their influence beyond title and position. The steps that foster authority are as follows:

1. Position: People follow your lead because they have to, however your influence does not extend beyond the lines of your job description.
2. Relationships: People follow your lead beyond your stated authority because they want to.
3. Results: People follow your lead because of what you have accomplished within the organization.
4. Reproduction: People follow your lead because of what you have helped them with. This is where long-term growth to the organization and its members occurs.
5. Respect: People follow your lead because of who you are and what you represent.

At each of these steps, remain aware that compliance sometimes hides in the wings. In Chapter 8 we discussed the importance of creating learning environments. A learning organization encourages people to develop personal mastery through commitment to a personal vision. Whereas a personal vision is tied to individualized learning, a shared vision facilitates organizational learning. Shared vision has *we* at its core: what do we want to create within the organization (Tohidi & Jabbari, 2012). However, it is through the development of an individualized vision that professionals excel and learn, not because they are told to, but because they want to. If individuals do not have their own vision, they simply sign up for someone else's. The result is compliance, never commitment.

In fact, real commitment is quite rare. Senge (2006) tells us that much of the time, what passes for commitment is compliance. *Commitment* describes the state of feeling fully responsible for making a vision happen and the creation of structures to support it. In some organizations there are relatively few people truly enrolled and even fewer committed. The great majority of individuals are in a state of compliance. Compliant followers go along with a vision and do what is expected of them. Often, compliance is confused with enrollment and commitment because compliance has prevailed for so long that it is difficult to recognize anything else. In addition, there are several levels of compliance and some of the behaviors look quite similar. A hierarchy of attitudes related to comittment looks something like this (Belasco & Stayer, 1993; Boldt, 1993; Papir-Bernstein, 1995):

- Apathy: Individuals are neither for nor against the vision. There is no expressed interest, enthusiasm, or energy and the person is basically waiting for the discussion to be over so that they can go home.
- Noncompliance: Individuals do not see any benefits of the vision, and will not do what is expected of them.
- Grudging compliance: Individuals do not see benefits, but do not want to lose a position, and so they do what is expected because they feel they have to. The individual does make it known, however, that they are not on board.
- Genuine compliance: Individuals do see the benefit of the vision, and do exactly what is expected but not one inch more. They follow "the letter of the law" and could be described as "good soldiers."
- Enrollment: Individuals totally buy into it and does whatever can be done to make it happen within "the spirit of the law."
- Commitment: Individuals create new laws and structures to insure that it happens. They do whatever it takes.

360-Degree Leadership, Collective Leadership, and Leadership Assessment

Kent McKamy (2018a) uses metaphors of other types of activities to describe effective 360-degree leadership. As a golfer, you cannot become successful by knowing only how to putt, or by being proficient with only one driver. In construction work, if the only tool you have access to is a hammer, every problem starts to look like a nail. The best leaders excel in all facets of leadership. According to McKamy (K. McKamy, personal communication, February 2, 2018), the Total Leader Concept is still considered a trend in leadership development, because it addresses 360-degree internal and external training.

Internal, or individualized, training targets personal productivity, personal leadership, motivational leadership, and strategic leadership. *Personal productivity* is the ability to manage yourself, your time, and your priorities to operate at maximum effectiveness. *Personal leadership* is the ability to be a leader in your own life, to determine what you want to be involved with, plan for it, make it happen, and self-evaluate your success. *Motivational leadership* is the ability to motivate others to express passion, act with enthusiasm, and inspire innovative actions and outcomes. *Strategic leadership* is the ability to lead an organization by developing strategies for optimizing vision and purpose. (K. McKamy, personal communication, February 2, 2018, 2018a).

Boundary-spanning leadership includes attention to leading in and from all directions. In a book by Matha and Boehm, it is reported that internal learning programs focus strongly on management and leadership skill-building (2008). The book described the importance of internal communications, as discussed in the previous chapter, and of listening to what is needed from the ground up. That reinforces the 360-degree leadership approach for creating a positive and productive work environment. Communications that revisit the organization's culture, values, policies, evaluations systems, and best practices have been an ongoing trend in the last several years. Another recurring theme in boundary-spanning leadership is understanding generational and gender diversity, and its impact on the perception of leadership and organizational hierarchy (Lamson, 2018).

For 360-degree leadership to be effective, organizations must know that they are not the hierarchies of the past, where one person had all leadership or management responsibilities. Decisions today are made following instant connections on email and messaging, and emojis have replaced vocal inflection and body language. Our workforce has more generations participating than ever before, and each generation has different values, attitudes, and beliefs.

A leadership consulting firm, The Human Factor (Wells, 2018), describes the future of leadership as driven by the need for greater agility, flexibility, and responsiveness to the diversity of workers and changing workplaces. Collective leadership and attention to generational diversity are two emerging trends. Teams, rather than a single individual, now tackle adaptive challenges in the workplace. The concept of collective leadership is certainly not new, but its current influence is fueled by generational styles and preferences. Millennials, in particular, are considered team-players whose exposure to technological innovation will certainly impact their leadership styles (Wells, 2018). Boss (2016) reports that top leadership trends in the last few years included encouraging more human interaction and prioritizing wellness plans. He also included more "we" and less "me," which focused on work teams, networks, knowledge sharing cultures, and cross-pollination. Another trend that keeps appearing is increased attention to curiosity, which sparks creativity, innovation, and growth potential.

The use of 360-degree leadership facilitates the need for a 360-degree assessment approach. Many companies use a 360-degree type of assessment to gather input about employees' performance not only from supervisors, but also from coworkers and the employees themselves. These types of assessments pinpoint areas for individual improvement and create a culture of learning and continuous improvement throughout the organizations. They incorporate input from all members of the organizational community (The Wallace Foundation [TWF], 2009). The work of leadership is no longer a solo activity, as traditional organizational boundaries seem to be dissolving. Our new work environments are characterized by increased levels of complexity and interconnectedness, which calls for involvement with boundary spanning, collaboration and network thinking.

Within the last ten years, greater attention has been focused on leadership assessment. Researchers from Vanderbilt University (Vanderbilt Assessment of Leadership in Education [VAL-ED], 2012) concluded that whereas leadership assessment topics are a mile in width, they are only an inch in depth. In other words, so many aspects of leadership can be assessed, but rarely is one aspect assessed in detail. Gone are the days when we assessed leadership with a single form or interview. Now, it is more often an ongoing process connected to the objective of continuous professional development and program improvement. The most important question is "What assessment processes will enhance leadership effectiveness in meeting organization mission and objectives?" Organizational leaders are the major impetus behind efforts for collaboration and cohesion around organizational goals, and the commitment to achieve those goals (Goldring, Porter, Murphy, Elliott, & Cravens, 2009; Razik & Swanson, 2010).

The assessment of leaders is not a new practice within schools and districts, and research by The Wallace Foundation examines assessment practices and trends. In the past, assessments focused on knowledge and traits, rather than behaviors and actions. Today, a key challenge for leader assessment is to narrow the focus to the most potent performance behaviors that can promote improvement in organizational outcomes as they relate to the people served (TWF, 2009).

The purpose of a leadership assessment is to gather information so that decisions can be made that affect individual leaders and the organizations they are part of. At best, the information will be adaptable to multiple purposes and contexts. For example, assessments can be used for summative and formative purposes. Summative purposes might include hiring and placement, and formative purposes would target individual and organizational improvement. In addition, assessments should be flexible enough to be utilized by leaders in different career stages (i.e., for novice as well as seasoned leaders; Goldring et al., 2009; Murphy, Elliot, Goldring, & Porter, 2010). When assessments are used to enhance individual performance and organizational accountability, they can be a driving factor in supporting and encouraging behaviors and skills that improve organizational leadership. Continuous improvement is the ultimate benefit of effective leadership assessment.

An assessment process that supports leadership needs to focus on "driver" behaviors, be anchored in leadership standards, promote organizational innovation, and lead to appropriate individual and organizational development (TWF, 2009). An assessment system can serve to align learning communities, accountability, and organizational expectations. The VAL-ED assessment tool (VAL-ED, 2012; Polikoff et al., 2009) identifies the following key activities of leadership that should be considered for assessment:

1. Planning: coherently discussing policies, practices and organizational procedures;

2. Implementing: engaging people, ideas and resources for actualizing necessary activities;
3. Supporting: creating conditions that facilitate the use of financial, political, technological and human resources;
4. Advocating: promoting the diverse needs of the organization and communities it serves;
5. Communicating: developing, utilizing and maintaining systems of communications exchange within all organizational communities;
6. Monitoring: systematically collecting and analyzing data to guide decisions and actions for continuous improvement.

Please see Appendix 9–A for an example of an assessment for organizational learning capacity.

The Spirit of Leadership

Today, there is increased interest in spirituality in many facets of life, including the workplace. Spirituality, and its integration with leadership in a variety of fields of service, is now a compelling issue for professionals in the management sector. Spiritual leadership theory has at its core the goal of organizational transformation by creating "value congruence across the strategic, empowered team, and individual levels to, ultimately, foster higher levels of organizational commitment, productivity, and employee well-being" (Fry, Vitucci, & Cedillo, 2005, p. 835). The concept of *workplace spirituality* is the simple idea that employees have an inner life that both nourishes and is nourished by meaningful work they perform within a community. The most prevalent type of leadership practice that integrates principles of spirit is called *servant leadership*. The essence of servant leadership is the notion that a leader's service to others is a fundamental and top priority that benefits all (Greasley & Bocarnea, 2014; Robinson et al., 2013).

Some might say that visionary leadership is in short supply today, largely because of society's value on material capital and corporate power. In order for leadership to inspire sustainable vision, it needs to pursue two other forms of capital: social capital and spiritual capital. Social capital manifests in trust, empathy, and commitment to the health of the organization. It is often measured by emotional intelligence (EI or EQ), discussed earlier in this chapter and in preceding chapters. Alternatively, spiritual capital reflects what an organization exists for, believes in, takes responsibility for, and aspires toward (Zohar, 2005). Zohar and Marshall talk about a third Q, *spiritual intelligence*, which is the intelligence with which we address and solve problems of meaning and value, place actions and lives in a wider and richer context, express creativity, sanctify everyday experience, and temper rigid rules with understanding and compassion (Zohar & Marshall, 2001; Papir-Bernstein, 2018). In her writings about leadership and corporate structures, Zohar describes the inter-related mental, emotional, and spiritual systems of operation and their relationship to healthy organizations (2005). Leaders can develop spiritual intelligence by attending to the following principles:

- Self-awareness: paying attention to your own motivations and values
- Vision and value: acting from principles of deep belief
- Holism: seeing larger patterns, connections and relationships
- Compassion: feel the distress of others
- Celebration of diversity: placing value on differences and uniqueness
- Ability to reframe: standing back and seeing other perspectives
- Sense of vocation: feeling called upon to serve and give back

Cobb, Puchalski, and Rumbold (2012) state, "the engagement of spirituality with health care can thus be seen as a core strategy for humanizing health care through its focus on inner meaning, approaches to suffering (and loss), and compassionate practice" (p. viii). As such, spirituality provides a perspective on, and orientation to, the world, a way of cultivating the mind, thinking about the soul, and a general way of life. Research involving attention to spiritual components of care is still in its infancy in our field, but on the rise. To explore the role of spirituality in professional practice, Spillers (2007, 2011) surveyed students, clients and practitioners regarding the inclusion of spirituality in treatment models and curricula. Over 70% of students and adult clients felt it was appropriate for SLPs to address spirituality.

Spirituality has been defined as the innate human need to find meaning in life and in experiences, as well as to connect with something larger than oneself. Although alternative health care practices have re-introduced Western health care to the body-mind-spirit perspective for health and healing, spirituality is just beginning to enter the formal lexicon of SLPs (Palmer, 2003; Papir-Bernstein, 2018; Winslow & Wehtje-Winslow, 2007). Mathisen and colleagues (2015) conducted a literature review of practitioners' acknowledgment of spirituality as part of their practice across a range of SLP practice areas, and identified only 15 published articles. The publications focused on three broad themes: holistic practice, patient-centered care, and cultural and linguistic diversity. The review revealed that holistic practices and patient-centered care are enhanced through SLPs' development of empathy, compassion, and rapport, as reflected by the clients' core beliefs. In addition, clients' core beliefs (including aspects of gratitude and spirituality) influenced their own behaviors and their expectations regarding treatment outcomes. Spiritual resources and beliefs also provide a means to help clients cope with grief, loss, and decision-making that can improve quality of life (Mathisen, 2010; Mathisen et al., 2015; Mathisen, Carey, & Threats, 2017; Papir-Bernstein, 2018).

Most training and professional development programs acknowledge the intersection of three domains: intellect (head), clinical skills (hands), and patient/practitioner affect (heart). The have also begun to acknowledge the conjunction of spirituality and health care, a fourth domain, with an understanding of spirituality as it relates to universality and inclusivity, rather than religiosity. This conjunction is historical, intellectual, and practical because at the intersection of spirituality and health care is concern for humans, which is the critical interest CSD practitioners have in health, healing, and response to situations that disrupt communicative abilities. Why should we include spirituality in our leadership programs and clinical practice approaches?

Mathisen and colleagues offer the following reasons worthy of consideration (Mathisen et al., 2015; Papir-Bernstein, 2018):

1. There is increasing evidence linking improved outcomes in health and wellness with attention to spirituality.
2. In Western culture, there is a return to the mind-body-spirit paradigm, and treating each separately may conflict with natural healing processes and health outcomes.
3. It reinforces the belief that people function as whole complex systems, and should not be viewed as an impaired body part or disability.
4. It ensures client-centered practice that is meaningful to the client, ethical, and respectful of culture and diversity.
5. It reinforces inclusive and family-centered practice because it considers family issues and cultural traditions.
6. It encourages self-awareness, mindfulness, and realistic expectations related to beliefs and practices that can inhibit or advance therapy.

Mindful Leadership

Mindfulness training is all the rage in leadership development circles, and one might certainly say it is trending. There is no question it is trending in our discipline, as a search on ASHA's website quickly unveils many articles and presentations in the last several years. In addition, at the 2017 ASHA Convention, Goldie Hawn presented a well-attended keynote speech about her educationally-based mindfulness program for children, called mindUP.

More and more employees are unwilling to accept purely top-down approaches in the workplace. In addition, more and more employees are looking for meaning, happiness and connectedness at work. Chapter 8 discussed attitudes about our own well-being, and that personal and professional happiness are driven by the same themes: making a difference, being useful, connecting with something greater, establishing balance, and wanting community (Papir-Bernstein, 2018). The new way of leading is a people-centered approach. Hougaard and Carter (2018) wrote about two leadership traits that are currently trending—mindfulness and compassion—and how to apply them in your leadership practice. The surveyed over 52,000 upper level managers and found that 86% rated themselves as inspirational and positive role models. However, this percentage stands in stark contrast to the 82% of employees who found their leaders uninspiring.

Mindful leadership engenders people-centered leadership. Mindful practices help us find focus, resilience, and greater self-awareness. Compassion facilitates understanding of people at an emotional level, and improves the way we lead ourselves, our employees, our students, and our organizations. Mindfulness training offers the very thing we all want more of in our personal and professional lives: space. Mental and emotional space enlarges our capacity to see, feel, hear, and reflect upon what is in front of us as well as inside of us. When we have space, we can deal with problems creatively and humanely, rather than from a perspective of pressure. Bottom line, we need to train ourselves to notice when we are on autopilot or distracted and to redirect our full attention to the task at hand. (Marturano, 2014). There are endless sources of information on this topic, however a good place to begin is simply by going to Janice Marturano's website (2018), *Finding the Space to Lead.*

Mindfulness training is not about taking deep breaths; it is not a religion or a behavior management program. It is a methodology that sometimes includes meditations, affirmations, reflections, and purposeful pauses. Mindfulness training and sustained practice can produce improvement in three key leadership capacities: resilience, collaboration, and agility. Reitz and Chaskalson (2016a, 2016b) conducted the world's first published study of a multisession mindful leader program. Their data was drawn from 57 business leaders who attended training workshops and participated in conference calls. The leaders were assigned home practice of meditations, affirmations, and other exercises. The study showed that best results were achieved when the training took place in conjunction with sustained practice using formal mindfulness exercises for at least 10 minutes a day. They offer some suggestions for establishing formal mindfulness as a daily practice:

- Choose a time when you are most likely to practice, such as first thing in the morning or right before bed. Make it a habit.
- Set realistic expectations for your practice.
- Notice the benefits of your practice.
- Connect with others who are interested in becoming more mindful.

Mindful practices are very much connected with reflective practices and both are important trends in business and education. They both foster problem-solving, decision-making, and critical thinking. Reflection begins with open-mindedness and assumption of responsibility, and evolves into a willingness to question our practices for the purpose of self-growth and improved outcomes for our employees, students, and clients. Reflection has potential to bridge theory with practice, balance science with client-centered care, link evidence-based practice with practice-based evidence, and contribute to the cultivation of ethical principles of leadership (Caty, Kinsella, & Doyle, 2016; Papir-Bernstein, 2018).

Stone-Goldman (2012) identified mindfulness, or focused attention, as one of our most productive reflective tools, and describes it as the conscious direction of our attention to our experiences. Mindful and reflective practices include a thoughtful consideration and questioning of what we do, what we say, what works, and what does not. The process begins with a willingness to self-examine (Papir-Bernstein, 2018). Mindfulness training has been proposed for SLP graduate students and continuing education programs for practitioners (Beck, Verticchio, Seeman, Milliken, & Schaab, 2017; Seikel et al., 2016). Please refer to Papir-Bernstein (2018, pp. 87–91) for a more complete discussion about mindfulness and its utilization in our field.

Remember, if you want to integrate mindfulness into your workplace as part of your leadership approach, begin with yourself. Develop your own personal practice on a daily basis. Allocate space for people to practice in the workplace, someplace private and quiet if possible. Encourage people to practice together. Consider beginning meetings with a mindful minute (Reitz & Chaskalson, 2016b).

Communities of Practice

In today's world of interconnectedness, people must all learn to work together in new ways. One of the ways that transformation occurs in leadership cultures is through the implementation of communities of practice (CoP). CoP enable people to connect and experience the spirit of learning, knowledge sharing, and collaboration for the purpose of individual, as well as organizational development. In such communities, members from all layers of an organization come together and discuss their visions and views about leadership. Motivations may differ. Some members of the community want to share their experiences, some want to become better leaders, some want to learn about leadership, and others want to implement their learning into arenas of practical experience. However, all CoP members have one thing in common—they are passionate about leadership. By exchanging information, sharing resources and relaying experiences, members learn from one another and create opportunities to develop professionally and personally.

From a conceptual perspective, CoP can be viewed as an outgrowth of social learning theory. According to Wenger's explanation of this theory (2003), learning occurs through active participation in practices of social communities. Such participation involves both a kind of action and a form of belonging (through interactions), and "shapes not only what we do, but also who we are and how we interpret what we do" (p. 4). It impacts our practices, our sense of community, whether we experience our work as meaningful, and our identity within the work environment.

Communities of practice are all around us. It is not unusual to belong to several at once, and they tend to shift and move around over the course of our lives. One of the challenges of forward-thinking leadership is to identify and sustain the interconnected CoP that already exist within an organization, and create the momentum and infrastructure to form new communities. In fact, CoP are the newest type of organizational structure for disseminating tacit knowledge through knowledge sharing and experiential exchanges. They can drive strategy, promote the implementation of best practices, facilitate organizational change, and help recruit and retain professional talent (Wenger & Snyder, 2000). The implementation of such communities in business, health care, and education is relatively new, however the concept is ancient. It can be traced back to ancient Greece and the formation of groups of workers dedicated to a common mission (referred to as societies, craftsmen, masons, and guilds). Members of these communities would guide, drive, motivate, and inspire the sharing of knowledge assets and expertise (Papir-Bernstein, 2018).

Communities of practice allow us to practice a very important professional skill—the ability to network. Network expansion can benefit us in so many ways, such as by increasing professional confidence. It provides people as resources so that when we have questions, we can call on someone with demonstrated expertise in a particular area of practice. Nothing feels better than going to a professional meeting or conference, and having people you know come over and greet you. Networking facilitates the likelihood of that happening.

One way to establish professional networks is to get involved with volunteer leadership. One of the most valuable coP is the collaboration between ASHA and the state speech-language-hearing associations (SSLHAs). ASHA supplies a state advocacy team liaison to facilitate communications on the state level, as well as additional state advocacy resources on their website (ASHA State Advocacy, n.d.-b). There is a State Action Toolkit, model bills to help craft legislation, and information about the three advocacy networks: SEALs (State Education Advocacy Leaders), StAMP (State Advocates for Medicare Policy) and STARs (State Advocates for Reimbursement). Information is available on each state's section of the ASHA website through the state advocacy link. The link includes contact information for regulatory and governmental agencies in each state, as well as information about licensure laws and teacher requirements. Both ASHA and your SSLHA can help you with recruitment, professional development, strategic planning, and information on state trends regarding licensure and policy changes.

Other ASHA communities include those for Special Interest Groups, committees and councils, specialty certification groups, and the latest one, the Leadership Academy (ASHA Leadership

Academy, n.d.-a). The Leadership Academy is open to all ASHA members through a simple registration process, and enables access to leadership assessments, webinars, discussions, and a resource library of articles, books, and videos. It was an outgrowth of the outstanding work accomplished by the Committee on Leadership Cultivation (CLC) and Leadership Nominations and Cultivation Board (LNCB) that began in 2013 and extends through the present time. We continue our discussion about leadership cultivation in the following section.

Leadership Cultivation

Leadership cultivation takes place in universities and professional associations all over the world. It all begins with civic engagement and service learning. One purpose of higher education is to help students develop reflective lives in preparation for "citizenship." Universities, by incorporating the valuable experience of service learning with other requirements, provide students and their professors with early exposure to a culture of partnership with professional and neighborhood associations. It helps participants develop soft skills, such as EI, raises the place of volunteering in society, supports needy organizations, and facilitates the development of active citizenship, which enriches our democracy and contributes to social cohesion and community (Papir-Bernstein, 2018). For a self-assessment in the area of EI, please see Appendix 9–B.

In the field of leadership, there is growing recognition that EI and organizational skills, as components of professional credibility, are as important as technical expertise and that the most vulnerable jobs in our upcoming robot economy involve tasks that are repetitive and more easily predictable, regardless of how much training they require. Professions that rely on creative thinking, emphasize empathy, and demand interpersonal communication are somewhat more protected (Ford, 2016).

One of the leading sources of information about employment of college graduates since the mid-1950s is the National Association of Colleges and Employers (NACE). Data collected over the last several decades tells us that employers considering new college graduates for job opening are looking for people with leadership capabilities. In addition, when employers were asked which attributes they look for on a candidate's resume, the most common response was "leadership" (77.8%) chose "leadership." The NACE (2013) also reports that leadership skills can make or break a hiring decision (National Association of Colleges and Employers, 2013). When employers are asked to choose between two equally qualified candidates, they often choose the one with experience in a leadership position (Papir-Bernstein, 2018).

Leadership sometimes begins with volunteer work. Volunteerism adds value to the health of associations and civic life in general. We know that volunteers allow organizations to expand their reach by broadening parameters such as age and diversity. However, there is still a gap in knowledge about volunteer motivation and management. A key findings from a 2008 study conducted by the American Society of Association Executives (ASAE) and the Center for Association Leadership, was that organizational strategies can support or discourage volunteering. The number one reason that members of professional associations did not volunteer was a lack of information about volunteer opportunities (Gazley & Dignam, 2008).

A 2016 ASHA leadership survey (ASHA Committee on Leadership Cultivation [CLC], 2016b) of more than 125 CSD academic program directors, found that 93% of program directors felt responsible for motivating their students to take on volunteer leadership roles. They reported that volunteer leadership roles included serving on a student association or organizing a campus for community events. Their top five reasons for promoting volunteer leadership were supporting and driving change, giving back to the professions, contributing to best practices, impacting our professional associations, and learning new skills. In the same survey (ASHA CLC, 2016a), the majority of program directors surveyed said that key areas of leadership are integrated into academic courses, practicum seminars, and clinical experiences. At least 70% of program directors confirmed that the following areas of leadership training were covered in their curricula: ethics, collaboration, critical thinking, advocacy, and problem-based learning. However, interestingly, only 45% of respondents had broached the topic of volunteer leadership with their students.

In 2013, a subcommittee of ASHA Ad Hoc Committee on CLC, 2013 surveyed over 930 volunteer and staff leaders (with a 43% response rate) about four topics: important leadership qualities; necessary content knowledge, strategies for leadership development, and commitment expectations of volunteer leaders. More than half (54%) of volunteer leaders reported that they got first involved with ASHA leadership because of a recruiter. Thirty-five percent said that they became involved through their own initiative. Another third (29%) indicated that their start evolved from experience with a state association or other professional organization.

There is no question that leadership cultivation and volunteer leadership are now on our professional radar, and ASHA has some excellent resources. On the website, if you search for *volunteer*, one of the results is the Become a Volunteer page. Scroll down to *Get Involved!* and you'll find links for where following opportunities (most with their own set of links) present themselves:

- Join a committee, board, or council (currently more than 35 standing committees)
- Volunteer as a writer (for information handouts, journals, online resources, etc.)
- Become a mentor (for various ASHA leadership or research programs)
- Become an ASHA member representative (with subject expertise or speaking engagements)
- Get involved with grassroots advocacy (with neighborhood groups, visiting Congress, etc.)
- Participate on a review panel (for grants, self-study programs, and awards)
- Assist with technology (assist with the practice portal, offer feedback on the website)
- Participate in a focus group (share experiences and information)
- Help with the accreditation process (conduct site visits, establish policies)

The Future of Leadership Practices

Nick Petrie of the Center for Creative Leadership (2014) led an interdisciplinary study, in collaboration with Harvard University, to examine the future of leadership practices and leadership development. His four areas of focus were leadership approaches, what works, what doesn't work, and where we are headed. The following four trends were identified: increased focus on vertical development, transfer of greater developmental ownership to the individual, collective rather than individual leadership, and innovation in leadership development approaches.

Development within an organization can be viewed as horizontal or vertical. Most organizations spend more time on horizontal development, viewed as competencies, skills, abilities and behaviors, usually transmitted from person to person. Horizontal development targets the acquisition of new knowledge, skills, abilities, and behaviors. Vertical development occurs in developmental stages, much like cognitive development, and must be earned. The current trend is to target a combination of vertical and horizontal development approaches. Petrie (2014) uses the metaphor of a glass of water to explain the difference between vertical horizontal development. With horizontal development, you pour water into a glass and the water represents leadership techniques. The glass will eventually fill up. In contrast, with vertical development you try to expand the glass itself, so that it has increased capacity to take in more content. Thus, the structure of the glass has been transformed. It is necessary to expand in both horizontal and vertical directions.

In addition to new skills and knowledge, a new expansive mindset is necessary to make the shift to network-centric, participatory, and collaborative leadership styles. Hackman (2002) reminds us that growth fuels growth, and that the workers who grow the most are the ones motivated to keep growing. In other words, the more growth we experience the more we want to experience. The implication is that if leaders help people get started on vertical development, their drive for greater growth will fuel the ongoing momentum as they build your team of teams.

Why is a team of teams important? Because leadership today is more of a collective endeavor than an individual endeavor. As a result, leaders must nurture environmental conditions needed for leadership to flourish among networks of professionals. To build your team of teams, you must transform your organization from traditional silos to a hybrid organizational model with its own operating rhythm. Fussell (2017) talks about this operating rhythm, and that "finding the cadence-based balance between the creation of shared consciousness and windows of empowered execution" is critical to success of a hybrid model of leadership (p. 5). He refers to expanding decision-making authority during periods of empowered execution to create decision space. Hybrid organizations balance horizontal networking and respect for organizational vertical hierarchies within the same structure.

Another trend in the future of leadership practices is the transfer of developmental ownership. We all tend to develop faster when we feel responsible for our own progress. This trend targets the individual owning their own development, rather than the organization assuming responsibility for the individual's growth. Theories of adult learning are led by constructivist and social theories, and suggest that active learning is best achieved by self-directed learners who have multiple opportunities to practice and gain experience, collaborate with others, participate with CoP, reflect upon their experiences, and formulate principles for practice based on their reflections.

Motivation to grow is highest when leaders feel a sense of autonomy over their own development. Self-directed learning is one of the most powerful principles in adult learning for several reasons. First, it relates to a larger concept called self-actualization, or sense of accomplishment. Second, it relates to a professional demand to keep up to date through lifelong learning and continuing education. And third, it allows learners to take responsibility for regulating and monitoring their own learning content and pace (Bandura, 1986; Harris, 2011; Papir-Bernstein, 2018).

Kegan and Lahey (2009) formulated four simple questions that inform ownership of development, and should be answerable by any individual in the organization:

1. What area of growth are you working on?
2. How are you working on it?
3. Who else knows and cares that you are working on it?
4. Why is this area of growth important?

Conclusion

Leaders in our profession need to be aware of new trends and discover ways to showcase innovations so that we can move the profession to new heights. Leadership is being redefined, moving from a person (in a role) to a network (within a shared process). The network involves anyone and everyone who is actively involved in producing direction, alignment, and commitment. The act of leadership is not necessarily tied to an individual, but distributed freely across boundaries and throughout networks of people. Leaders must consider how best to have leadership flourish in their organization by creating a leadership culture that supports the open flow of information, flexible hierarchies, and distributed decision-making (Hackman, 2002; McCauley & Van Velsor, 2004; Petrie, 2014).

Moving out of individual silos provides opportunities to improve interprofessional practice outcomes by coordinating services and learning from one another (Pickering & Embry, 2013). Leaders within organizations that become silo-spanning networks will at times find themselves fighting off the ghosts of outdated bureaucratic norms and routines. Fussell (2017) takes us through a discussion of where those ghosts come from, beginning with psychiatrist Carl Jung's explanation of collective unconscious archetypes. These archetypes are universal models that have existed since ancient times that conjure up steadfast definitions of concepts, which remain ingrained in our minds and become part of our intuitive understanding. Such is the case with leadership, and what leadership should look like. The exemplar is reflected in legend and has fueled a leader as hero mythology: the success of an organization is due to the efforts of one leader, the savior, the hero, the knower of all answers.

Because leadership is a collective process spread throughout networks of people, leaders need to contemplate conditions needed for leadership to flourish in their organization. This trend requires a transition to collective leadership speeding throughout the organizational networks, rather than residing within individual managers. Today's leaders are different. They align and empower teams, they pull diverse voices into the conversation, they decentralize decision-making, they model humility, they are servants to a common mission. Today's leaders are willing to shift their own identities by creating context for others to develop greatness and enhance the professional community (Manville, 2017). Today's leaders are willing to say to their organization:

> I understand the complexity of the environment. I understand that you must move faster than our structures allow for and that you understand your problems better than I ever could. I will create spaces for you to organically communicate and share information. I will empower you to make decisions and execute. I can help guide us on the path. (Fussell, 2017, p. 248)

Experiential Commentary

I have always enjoyed bringing fresh perspectives into my work by applying knowledge from many different disciplines, as well as my real-world experiences. Without realizing it, I had developed a trending style much like the trend forecaster Faith Popcorn. Perhaps her book influenced me in the early 1990's more than I realized. I continue to engage in some of the activities she suggests to keep a finger on the pulse of cultural trends; I scan best sellers, and buy an assortment of books for browsing. Yes, I still do prefer reading books, and all of those colored post-its I pick up at conventions come in handy for my notations. I use movies to illustrate teaching points in my classes, and pay close attention to the memes currently in favor. I also read trade magazines from other disciplines and talk with friends about current trends in their industries.

One day in a doctor's office, I picked up a fishing magazine. One article in a June issue talked about the importance of planning and implementing goals within the fishing process. There was an acronym used that really caught my eye, SMART, which stood for specific, measurable, attainable, relevant, and timely. I read the entire article and was struck at how applicable this concept was to our work. I tore it out, talked about it in my classes, and in September of that year was happy to discover that other professionals were paying attention to interdisciplinary messages. Someone had actually published an article about the same acronym in *The ASHA Leader.*

Reflective Questions

1. What motivated you to assume a leadership role, and what is your vision with respect to organizational leadership?
2. What techniques do you use for trend tracking?
3. What involvements have you had with generation-speak, and how have your leadership style and methodologies shifted as a result?
4. What specific changes in the clinical and educational landscapes have impacted your implementation of leadership principles?
5. How have you enhanced your individual and organizational value?
6. Describe your experiences with boundary-spanning 360-degree leadership? How might your past experiences impact your actions in the future?
7. Explain why and how mindful and reflective practices have assumed a place in the field.

References

Altran, S. (2001). The trouble with memes: Inference versus imitation in cultural creation. *Human Nature, 12*(4), 351–381.

Ad Hoc Committee on Reframing the Professions. (2013). *Final Report: Reframing the professions of speech-language pathology and audiology. ASHA.org.* Retrieved from http://www.asha.org/uploadedFiles/Reframing-the-Professions-Report.pdf

American Society of Association Executives (ASAE) and the Center for Association Leadership. (2008). *Designing your future: Key trends, challenges, and choices facing association and nonprofit leaders.* Washington, DC: Author.

American Speech-Language-Hearing Association (ASHA). (n.d.-a). *Leadership Academy.* Retrieved from https://community.asha.org/ leadershipacademy/home

American Speech-Language-Hearing Association (ASHA). (n.d.-b). *State Advocacy.* Retrieved from http://www.asha.org/advocacy/state/

American Speech-Language-Hearing Association (ASHA). (2017a). *Strategic pathway to excellence.* Retrieved from http://www.asha.org/ About/Strategic-Pathway/

American Speech-Language-Hearing Association (ASHA). (2017b). *Market trends.* Retrieved from https://www.asha.org/Careers/Market-Trends/

American Speech-Language-Hearing Association (ASHA). (2017c). ASHA members span 5 generations, 7 decades. *The ASHA Leader, 22,* 30. doi:10.1044/leader.AAG.22122017.30

Argyis, C., & Schon, D. (1996). *Organizational learning II: Theory, method, and practice.* Reading, MA: Addison-Wesley.

ASHA Ad Hoc Committee on Leadership Cultivation (CLC). (2013). *Final report.* Retrieved from http://www.asha.org/uploadedFiles/ Report-Ad-Hoc-Committee-on-Leadership-Cultivation.pdf

ASHA Committee on Leadership Cultivation (CLC). (2016a). CSD programs report widespread leadership coverage across curricula. *The ASHA Leader, 21,* 26.

ASHA Committee on Leadership Cultivation (CLC). (2016b). Why CSD programs encourage volunteer leadership. *The ASHA Leader, 21,* 28.

Bandura, A. (1986). *Social foundations of thought and action: A social cognitive theory.* Englewood Cliffs, NJ: Prentice Hall.

Beck, A. R., Verticchio, H., Seeman, S., Milliken, E., & Schaab, H. (2017). A mindfulness practice for communication sciences and disorders undergraduate and speech-language pathology graduate students: Effects on stress, self-compassion, and perfectionism. *American Journal of Speech-Language Pathology, 26,* 893–907.

Belasco, J. A., & Stayer, R. C. (1993). *Flight of the buffalo: Soaring to excellence and learning to let employees lead.* New York, NY: Warner Books

Boldt, S. G. (1993). *Zen and the art of making a living.* New York, NY: Penguin Group.

Boss, J. (2016, December 20). Be better prepared for 2017 with these 8 leadership trend projections. *Forbes Magazine.* Retrieved from https://www.forbes.com/sites/jeffboss/2016/12/20/be-better-pre pared-for-2017-with-these-8-leadership-trend-projections/

Bradberry, T., & Greaves, J. (2012). *Leadership 2.0.* San Diego, CA: TalentSmart.

Caty, M., Kinsella, E. A., & Doyle, P. C. (2016). Reflective practice in speech-language pathology: Relevance for practice and education.

Canadian Journal of Speech-Language Pathology and Audiology, *40*(1), 81–91.

Charan, R., Drotter, S., & Noel, J. (2000). *The leadership pipeline.* San Francisco, CA: Jossey-Bass.

Cobb, M., Puchalski, C., & Rumbold, B. (Eds.). (2012). *Oxford textbook of spirituality in healthcare.* New York, NY: Oxford University Press.

Combi, C. (2015). *Generation Z: Their voices, their lives.* London, UK: Hutchinson.

Cook, B. G., Cook, L., & Landrum, T. J. (2013). Moving research into practice: Can we make dissemination stick? *Council for Exceptional Children, 79*(2), 163–180.

Drucker, P. F. (1999). *Management challenges for the 21st century.* New York, NY: Harper Business.

Edgar, G. (2004). *Classics on fractals.* Boulder, CO: Westview Press.

Ernst, C., & Chrobot-Mason, D. (2010). *Boundary spanning leadership: Six practices for solving problems, driving innovation, and transforming organizations.* New York, NY: McGraw-Hill Professional.

Finney, M. I. (2013). *The truth about getting the best from people.* Upper Saddle River, NJ: Pearson Education.

Ford, M. (2016). *Rise of the robots: Technology and the threat of a jobless future.* New York, NY: Basic Books.

Fry, L. W., Vitucci, S., & Cedillo, M. (2005). Spiritual leadership and army transformation: Theory, measurement, and establishing a baseline. *The Leadership Quarterly, 16,* 835–862.

Fussell, C. (2017). *One mission: How leaders build a team of teams.* New York, NY: Portfolio/Penguin.

Gazley, B., & Dignam, M. (2008). *The decision to volunteer.* Washington, DC: ASAE & The Center for Association Leadership.

Goldring, E., Porter, A., Murphy, J., Elliott, S. N., & Cravens, X. (2009). Assessing learning-centered leadership: Connections to research, professional standards, and current practices. *Leadership and Policy in Schools 8,* 1–36.

Greasley, P. E., & Bocarnea, M. C. (2014). The relationship between personality type and the servant leadership characteristic of empowerment. *Procedia-Social and Behavioral Sciences, 124,* 11–19. https://doi.org/10.1016/j.sbspro.2014.02.454

Hackman, R. R. (2002). *Leading teams: Setting the stage for great performances.* Cambridge, MA: Harvard Business Press.

Harris, I. B. (2011). Conceptions and theories of learning for workplace education. In J. P. Hafler (Ed.), *Extraordinary learning in the workplace.* (pp. 39–62). New York, NY: Springer.

Heath, C., & Heath, D. (2007). *Made to stick.* New York, NY: Random House.

Hendrix, J. S. (2005). *Aesthetics & the philosophy of spirit*. New York, NY: Peter Lang.

Hildreth, P., & Kimble, C. (2002). *The duality of knowledge*. *Information Research*, *8*(1), 1–18. Retrieved from http://InformationR.net/ir/8-1/paper142.html

Hougaard, R., & Carter, J. (2018). *The mind of the leader*. Watertown, MA: Harvard Business Review Press.

Kamhi, A. G. (2004). A meme's eye view of speech-language pathology. *Language Speech-Hearing Services in the Schools*, *3*, 105–111.

Kegan, R., & Lahey, L. (2009). *Immunity to change: How to overcome it and unlock potential in yourself and your organization*. Boston, MA: Harvard Business School Press.

KnowledgeWorks Forecast 4.0. (2018). *What's next for education changemaking?* Retrieved from https://knowledgeworks.org/wp-content/uploads/2018/01/shaping-education-changemakers-info graphic-1117.pdf

Lamson, M. (2018, January 3). The leadership development trends in 2018. *Inc.com*. Retrieved from https://www.inc.com/melissa-lam son/top-learning-development-trends-for-2018.html

Leal, A., & Roldan, J. (2001). Benchmarking and knowledge management. *OR Insight*, *14*(4), 11–22.

Lemke, A., & Dublinske, S. (2010). *Designing ASHA's future: Trends for the association and the professions*. Unpublished paper.

Lemke, A., & Dublinske, S. (2011). Forecasting the future: Impact of societal trends on the professions and ASHA. *The ASHA Leader*, *16*, 28–28.

Manville, B. (2017, June 28). How to be a horizontal and vertical leader at the same time. *Forbes Magazine*. Retrieved from https://www.forbes.com/sites/brookmanville/2017/06/28/how-to-be-a-horizon tal-and-vertical-leader-at-the-same-time/#49f453ba5bed

Marturano, J. (2014). *Finding the space to lead: A practical guide to mindful leadership*. New York, NY: Bloomsbury Press.

Marturano, J. (2018). Meditations & reflections. *FindingTheSpaceToLead.com*. Retrieved from https://findingthespacetolead.com/meditations-reflections/

Matha, B., & Boehm, M. (2008). *Beyond the babble: Leader communication that drives results*. Hoboken, NJ: Wiley.

Mathisen, B. (2010). *Including spirituality in speech pathology practice: A pilot study of undergraduates* [Unpublished manuscript]. The University of Newcastle, Department of Speech Pathology, New South Wales, UK.

Mathisen, B., Carey, L. B., Carey-Sargeant, C. L., Webb, G., Millar, C., & Krikheli, L. (2015). Religion, spirituality and speech-language pathology. *Journal of Religion and Health*, *54*(6), 2309–2323.

Mathisen, B. A., Carey, L. B., & Threats, T. T. (2017, November). *Holistic care: Speech-language pathology & spirituality*. Seminar presented at ASHA Convention, Los Angeles, CA.

Maxwell, J. C. (2011). *The 360 degree leader: Developing your influence from anywhere in the organization*. Nashville, TN: Thomas Nelson.

McCauley, C., & Van Velsor, E. (2004). *The Center for Creative Leadership handbook of leadership development*. San Francisco, CA: Jossey-Bass.

McKamy, K. (2018a). Atlantic Leadership Group: The Total Leader. Retrieved from http://www.atlanticleadershipgroup.com

McNeilly, L. (2018). Why we need to practice at the top of the license. *The ASHA Leader, 23*, 10–11.

Murphy, J., Elliott, S. N., Goldring, E., & Porter, A. C. (2010). Leaders for productive schools. In E. Baker, P. Peterson, & B. McGaw (Eds.), *International encyclopedia of education* (3rd ed., pp. 746–751). Oxford, UK: Elsevier.

National Association of Colleges and Employers (NACE). (2013). *NACE's professional competencies for college and university career services practitioners*. Retrieved from http://www.naceweb.org/career-development/standards-competencies/naces-professional-competencies-for-college-and-university-career-services-practitioners/

O'Dell, C., & Grayson, C. J. (1998). *If only we knew what we know: The transfer of internal knowledge and best practice*. New York, NY: The Free Press.

Palmer, P. J. (2003). Teaching with heart and soul: Reflections on spirituality in teacher education. *Journal of Teacher Education, 54*(5), 376–385.

Papir-Bernstein, W. (1995). *Supervision for the 21st century: Facilitating self-directed professional growth*. Seminar presented at New York State Speech-Language-Hearing Association (NYSSLHA), New York, NY.

Papir-Bernstein, W. (2012a). The artistry of practice-based evidence (PBE): One practitioner's path—Part I. In R. Goldfarb (Ed.), *Translational speech-language pathology and audiology* (pp. 51–57). San Diego, CA: Plural.

Papir-Bernstein, W. (2012b). The artistry of practice-based evidence (PBE): One practitioner's path—Part II. In R. Goldfarb (Ed.), *Translational speech-language pathology and audiology* (pp. 83–89). San Diego, CA: Plural.

Papir-Bernstein, W. (2018). *The practitioner's path in speech-language pathology: The art of school-based practice*. San Diego, CA: Plural.

Petrie, N. (2014). Future trends in leadership development [White paper]. *Center for Creative Leadership*. Retrieved from https://www.ccl.org/wp-content/uploads/2015/04/futureTrends.pdf

Pickering, J., & Embry, E. (2013). So long, silos. *The ASHA Leader, 18,* 38–45.

Polikoff, M. S., May, H., Porter, A. C., Elliott, S. N., Goldring, E., & Murphy, J. (2009). An examination of differential item functioning in the Vanderbilt Assessment of Leadership in Education. *Journal of School Leadership, 19*(6), 661–679.

Popcorn, F. (1991). *The Popcorn report: Faith Popcorn on the future of your company, your world, your life.* New York, NY: Doubleday.

Porter, M. (2010). What is value in health care? *New England Journal of Medicine, 363,* 2477–2481.

Rao, P. R. (2014, November). *Healthcare reform: Leading change as shift happens.* Short course presented at ASHA Convention, Orlando, FL.

Razik, T. A., & Swanson, A. D. (2010). *Fundamental concepts of educational leadership and management* (3rd ed.). Boston, MA: Allyn & Bacon.

Reitz, M., & Chaskalson, M. (2016a, November 4). Mindfulness works but only if you work at it. *Harvard Business Review.* Retrieved from https://hbr.org/2016/11/mindfulness-works-but-only-if-you-work-at-it

Reitz, M., & Chaskalson, M. (2016b, December 1). How to bring mindfulness to your company's leadership. *Harvard Business Review.* Retrieved from https://hbr.org/2016/12/how-to-bring-mindfulness-to-your-companys-leadership

Robinson, T. L., Papir-Bernstein, W., Chabon, S. S., Diefendorf, A. O., Franklin, T. C., Lubinsky, J., . . . Falzarano, A. (2013, November). *Leadership: It's more than a position.* Seminar presented at ASHA Convention, Chicago, IL.

Roger, D., & Petrie, N. (2017). *Work without stress: Building a resilient mindset for lasting success.* Colorado Springs, CO: Center for Creative Leadership.

Roseberry-McKibbin, C. (2017). Generation Z rising. *The ASHA Leader, 22,* 36–38. Retrieved from http://leader.pubs.asha.org/article.aspx?articleid=2664620

Seikel, T., Holst, J., Hudock, D., Ament, R., O'Donnell, J., Guryan, B., . . . Hatzenbuehler, L. (2016, November). *The mindful practitioner: Incorporating mindfulness into classroom, supervision and clinic.* Seminar presented at ASHA Conference, Philadelphia, PA.

Senge, P. (2006). *The fifth discipline: The art and practice of learning.* New York, NY: Doubleday.

Smith, E. A. (2001). The role of tacit and explicit knowledge in the workplace. *Journal of Knowledge Management, 5*(4), 311–321.

Spillers, C. S. (2007). An existential framework for understanding the counseling needs of clients. *American Journal of Speech-Language Pathology, 16,* 191–197.

Spillers, C. S. (2011). Spiritual dimensions of the clinical relationship. In R. F. Fourie (Ed.), *Therapeutic processes for communication disorders: A guide for students and clinicians* (pp. 229–243). East Sussex, UK: Psychology Press.

Stone-Goldman, J. (2012, November). *Reflective practice for emotional balance in professional relationships.* Paper presented at ASHA Convention, Atlanta, GA.

The Wallace Foundation (TWF). (2009). *Assessing the effectiveness of school leaders: New directions and new processes.* Retrieved from https://www.wallacefoundation.org/knowledge-center/pages/assessing-the-effectiveness-of-school-leaders.aspx

Tohidi, H., & Jabbari, M. M. (2012). Measuring organizational learning capacity. *Procedia: Social and Behavioral Sciences, 31,* 428–432. https://doi.org/10.1016/j.sbspro.2011.12.079

Vanderbilt Assessment of Leadership in Education (VAL-ED). (2012). Retrieved from https://valed.ioeducation.com

Wells, M. (2018). *Six future leadership trends.* The Human Factor Website. Retrieved from http://thehumanfactor.biz/six-future-leadership-trends/

Wenger, E. (2003). *Communities of practice: Learning, meaning, and identity.* New York, NY: Cambridge University Press.

Wenger, E., & Snyder, W. (2000, January–February). Communities of practice: The organizational frontier. *Harvard Business Review.* Retrieved from https://hbr.org/2000/01/communities-of-practice-the-organizational-frontier

Winslow, G. R., & Wehtje-Winslow, B. J. (2007). Ethical boundaries of spiritual care. *Medical Journal of Australia, 186*(10), 63–66.

Yip, J., Ernst, C., & Campbell, M. (2016). *Boundary spanning leadership: Mission critical perspectives from the executive suite.* Retrieved from https://www.ccl.org/wp-content/uploads/2015/04/BoundarySpanningLeadership.pdf

Ziskin, I. (2011). *WillBe: 13 reasons willbe's are luckier than wannabe's.* Sag Harbor, NY: EXec EXcel Group.

Ziskin, I. (2015). *Three: The human resources emerging executive.* Hoboken, NJ: Wiley.

Ziskin, I. (2016). The ten inflection points of coaching: Navigating the successful leadership coaching journey. In M. Finney (Ed.), *HR directions: HR leading lights on what you should know right now about leadership, engagement, technology, and growing your own world-class HR career* (pp. 14–153). Woodbridge, CA: HR C-Suite.

Zohar, D. (2005). Spiritually intelligent leadership. *Leader to Leader, 38,* 45–49. https://doi.org/10.1002/ltl.153

Zohar, D., & Marshall, I. (2001). *Spiritual intelligence: The ultimate intelligence.* New York, NY: Bloomsbury.

Organizational Learning Capacity

Wendy Papir-Bernstein (Adapted from Tohidi & Jabbari, 2012)

The following survey assesses fundamental and strategic elements of a learning organization. Please rate your level of agreement with the following statements using the following scale:

1 Strongly disagree, **2** Disagree,
3 Neither agree nor disagree, **4** Agree, **5** Strongly agree

I experience the organizational learning capacity in the following ways:

1. Open discussions about learning projects are encouraged.

   1   2   3   4   5

2. There is dedication to the change process when discussing mission and vision.

   1   2   3   4   5

3. I am aware of organization goals.

   1   2   3   4   5

4. I am encouraged to contribute to decision-making.

   1   2   3   4   5

5. I am encouraged to contribute professional development ideas.

   1   2   3   4   5

6. I am encouraged to question and offer suggestions for policy changes.

   1   2   3   4   5

7. We improve our work process by experimentation.

   1   2   3   4   5

8. Creative and innovative ideas are acknowledged and rewarded.

1   2   3   4   5

9. We have a system for learning from other similar organizations.

1   2   3   4   5

Reference

Tohidi, H., & Jabbari, M. M. (2012). Measuring organizational learning capacity. *Procedia--Social and Behavioral Sciences, 31*, 428–432. https://doi.org/10.1016/j.sbspro.2011.12.079

APPENDIX 9–B
The Emotional Competency Questionnaire

Wendy Papir-Bernstein (Adapted from Goleman, 1998)

The following survey assesses emotional competency related to personal competence (self-awareness, self-regulation, and motivation) and social competence (empathy and social skills). Please rate and circle your competency for each question, with **1** being a strong no and **5** being a strong yes.

Personal Competence (how we manage ourselves)

I. Self-Awareness (knowing your internal states, preferences, resources, and intuition)

A. *Emotional Awareness (recognizing your emotions and their effects)*

1. Do you know what you are feeling and why?

    1   2   3   4   5

2. Do you realize the connections between your feeling and what you think and say?

    1   2   3   4   5

3. Do you recognize how your emotions affect your performance?

    1   2   3   4   5

B. *Accurate Self-Assessment (knowing your strengths and weaknesses)*

1. Are you aware of your strengths and weaknesses?

    1   2   3   4   5

2. Are you reflective and do you learn from experience?

   1   2   3   4   5

3. Are you open to feedback, new perspectives, and self-development?

   1   2   3   4   5

C. *Self-Confidence (sureness about your self-worth and capabilities)*

1. Do you present yourself with self-assurance?

   1   2   3   4   5

2. Can you voice and defend views that are unpopular?

   1   2   3   4   5

3. Are you able to make sound decisions despite uncertainties and pressures?

   1   2   3   4   5

II. Self-Regulation (managing your internal states, impulses, and resources)

A. *Self-Control (managing disruptive emotions and impulses)*

1. Do you manage your impulsive feelings and distressing emotions well?

   1   2   3   4   5

2. Do you stay composed and positive even in trying moments?

   1   2   3   4   5

3. Do you think clearly and stay focused under pressure?

   1   2   3   4   5

B. *Trustworthiness (maintaining standards of honesty and integrity)*

1. Do you act ethically?

    1   2   3   4   5

2. Do you build trust through your reliability and authenticity?

    1   2   3   4   5

3. Do you admit your own mistakes?

    1   2   3   4   5

C. *Conscientiousness (taking responsibility for personal performance)*

1. Do you meet commitments and keep promises?

    1   2   3   4   5

2. Do you hold yourself accountable for meeting your objectives?

    1   2   3   4   5

3. Are you organized and careful in your work?

    1   2   3   4   5

D. *Adaptability (flexibility in handling change)*

1. Do you smoothly handle multiple demands and shifting priorities?

    1   2   3   4   5

2. Do you adapt your responses and strategies to fit changing circumstances?

    1   2   3   4   5

3. Are you flexible in how you view actions and events?

    1   2   3   4   5

E. *Innovativeness (being comfortable with and open to new ideas)*

1. Do you seek out fresh ideas from a wide variety of sources?

    1   2   3   4   5

2. Do you entertain original solutions to problems?

    1   2   3   4   5

3. Do you generate new ideas and take fresh perspectives?

    1   2   3   4   5

III. Motivation (emotional tendencies that facilitate reaching goals)

A. *Achievement Drive (striving to improve or meet standards of excellence)*

1. Are you results-oriented?

    1   2   3   4   5

2. Do you set challenging goals and take calculated risks?

    1   2   3   4   5

3. Do you pursue information and learn how to improve your performance?

    1   2   3   4   5

B. *Commitment (aligning with goals of the group or organization)*

1. Do you make personal or group sacrifices to meet a larger organizational goal?

    1   2   3   4   5

2. Do you find a sense of purpose in the larger mission?

    1   2   3   4   5

3. Do you actively seek out opportunities to fulfill the group's mission?

1   2   3   4   5

C. *Initiative (readiness to act on opportunities)*

1. Do you pursue goals beyond what is required or expected of you?

1   2   3   4   5

2. Do you cut through red tape and bend the rules when necessary to get the job done?

1   2   3   4   5

3. Do you mobilize others through unusual and enterprising efforts?

1   2   3   4   5

D. *Optimism (persistence in pursuing goals despite obstacles and setbacks)*

1. Do you persist in spite of setbacks?

1   2   3   4   5

2. Do you operate from hope of success rather than fear of failure?

1   2   3   4   5

3. Do you see setbacks as circumstance rather than personal flaws?

1   2   3   4   5

Social Competence (how we handle relationships)

I. Empathy (awareness of others' feelings, needs, and concerns)

A. *Understanding Others (taking an active interest in others' perspectives and concerns)*

1. Are you attentive to emotional cues and do you listen well?

   1   2   3   4   5

2. Do you show sensitivity and understand others' perspectives?

   1   2   3   4   5

3. Do you help out based on understanding other people's needs and feelings?

   1   2   3   4   5

B. *Developing Others (sensing what others need in order to bolster their abilities)*

1. Do you acknowledge and reward people's strengths and accomplishments?

   1   2   3   4   5

2. Do you offer useful feedback?

   1   2   3   4   5

3. Do you mentor and give timely coaching?

   1   2   3   4   5

C. *Service Orientation (anticipating, recognizing, and meeting the needs of others)*

1. Do you understand needs and match them to your services and products?

   1   2   3   4   5

2. Do you seek ways to increase satisfaction and loyalty?

     1   2   3   4   5

3. Do you offer appropriate assistance?

     1   2   3   4   5

D. *Leveraging Diversity (cultivating opportunities with diverse people)*

1. Do you respect and relate well to people from varied backgrounds?

     1   2   3   4   5

2. Do you understand diverse views and are you sensitive to group differences?

     1   2   3   4   5

3. Do you create environments where diverse people can thrive?

     1   2   3   4   5

E. *Political Awareness (reading a group's power relationships)*

1. Do you accurately read key power relationships?

     1   2   3   4   5

2. Do you detect crucial social networks?

     1   2   3   4   5

3. Do you understand the forces that shape people's views and actions?

     1   2   3   4   5

II. Social Skills (adeptness at facilitating desirable responses in others)

A. *Influence (using effective tactics for persuasion)*

1. Do you fine-tune presentations to appeal to the listener?

   1   2   3   4   5

2. Do you use strategies to build consensus and support?

   1   2   3   4   5

3. Do you orchestrate events to effectively make a point?

   1   2   3   4   5

B. *Communication (sending clear and convincing messages)*

1. Do you listen well, seek mutual understanding, and welcome shared information?

   1   2   3   4   5

2. Do you foster open communication and stay receptive to bad, as well as good news?

   1   2   3   4   5

3. Do you deal with difficult issues straightforwardly?

   1   2   3   4   5

C. *Conflict management (negotiating and resolving disagreements)*

1. Do you handle difficult people and tense situations with diplomacy and tact?

   1   2   3   4   5

2. Do you spot potential conflict and help de-escalate?

   1   2   3   4   5

3. Do you orchestrate win-win solutions?

1   2   3   4   5

D. *Leadership (inspiring and guiding groups and people)*

1. Do you arouse enthusiasm for a shared vision and mission?

1   2   3   4   5

2. Do you step forward to lead as needed, regardless of position?

1   2   3   4   5

3. Do you lead by example?

1   2   3   4   5

E. *Change Catalyst (initiating or managing change)*

1. Do you recognize the need for change and remove barriers?

1   2   3   4   5

2. Do you enlist others in the pursuit of change?

1   2   3   4   5

3. Do you model the change expected of others?

1   2   3   4   5

F. *Building Bonds (nurturing instrumental relationships)*

1. Do you cultivate and maintain extensive informal networks?

1   2   3   4   5

2. Do you seek out relationships that are mutually beneficial?

1   2   3   4   5

3. Do you build rapport and keep others in the loop?

1   2   3   4   5

G. *Collaboration and Cooperation (working with others toward shared goals)*

1. Do you balance focus on task with attention to relationships?

1   2   3   4   5

2. Do you share plans, information, and resources?

1   2   3   4   5

3. Do you spot and nurture opportunities for collaboration?

1   2   3   4   5

H. *Team Capabilities (creating group synergy in pursuing collective goals)*

1. Do you model team qualities like respect, helpfulness, and cooperation?

1   2   3   4   5

2. Do you build team identity and commitment?

1   2   3   4   5

3. Do you protect the group and share credit?

1   2   3   4   5

References

Goleman, D. (1998). *Working with emotional intelligence.* New York, NY: Bantam Books.

Papir-Bernstein, W. (2018). *The practitioner's path in speech-language pathology: The art of school-based practice.* San Diego, CA: Plural.

10

Mentoring Emerging Leaders

Regina Lemmon-Bush

The single biggest way to impact an organization is to focus on leadership development. There is almost no limit to the potential of an organization that recruits good people, raises them up as leaders and continually develops them.

—John Maxwell

Learning Objectives

The reader will learn:

- about the different leadership styles and how they influence mentoring and coaching.
- how to develop the knowledge and skills to mentor emerging leaders.
- how to interact with emerging leaders who may be of a different generation, culture, ethnicity, age, or sexual orientation.
- strategies to encourage leadership development in emerging leaders.
- about organizational silence and the role it plays in hindering organizational development.

Introduction

Mentoring emerging leaders can be rewarding for an experienced leader and beneficial to the longevity and success of an organization. Mentoring emerging leaders in clinically-based health care professions is most effective when an experienced leader has participated in a leadership development program (ASHA, 2013). Leadership teaches experienced leaders strategies for effective mentorship and how to avoid some of the pitfalls that may accompany the mentoring process. Emerging leaders benefit from the expertise of experienced leaders who can assist them by gradually transitioning emerging leaders into leadership positions; providing continuity and a seamless transfer of leadership within an organization. Continuity benefits the emerging leader by equipping and empowering them to meet the professional demands of the leadership position. The experienced and emerging leaders both experience a sense of success while the organization benefits by gaining a leader who will inspire employees to greatness, as opposed to a manager who guides every task. Mentoring, combined with leadership development, cultivates potential leaders and molds them into individuals who evolve into leadership positions, which positively impacts the organization and profession. Mentees (emerging leaders) enter leadership positions with a personal mission, vision, and strategic plan to lead others within an organization.

Acquiring Knowledge of Leadership Styles to Positively Impact Mentoring Relationships

There are several leadership styles, models, and theories, and each has the potential to impact an organization or mentoring relationship differently (Walston, 2017). Prior to becoming a mentor, individuals should learn about and reflect on their personal leadership style in order to positively impact the mentoring relationship. Similarly, knowledge of the varying styles of leadership should be shared with emerging leaders so they can learn the different styles while developing their own leadership style. This process not only helps transform individual emerging leaders, but also has the potential to (a) transform the type of leaders cultivated in Communication Sciences and Disorders (CSD), (b) increase work productivity, (c) positively impact the quality of the services provided to consumers, and (d) help increase job satisfaction, thereby retaining stellar employees. In turn, the mentor-mentee relationship and bond between the experienced and emerging leader becomes stronger. It is very important for emerging leaders to learn about leadership styles during the mentoring process so that they will consider their own leadership styles. When mentoring is most effective, mentors eventually become trusted colleagues and possibly friends.

Walston (2017) delineates the various leadership styles and models in the text *Organizational Behavior and Theory in Healthcare*. The summary of leadership theories and models in Table 10–1 can help experienced leaders understand how leadership functions to positively or negatively impact an organization.

As an experienced leader, reflect upon the key style factors delineated in Table 10–1 to assess your leadership skills and to share your knowledge of leadership models and styles with emerging leaders. Consider your personal experiences as an experienced leader and answer the following questions about your own leadership model and style as a means of engaging your mentee:

- Which best describe you?
- How has it affected your subordinates? Think of specific examples.
- Which are the best in your opinion? Why?
- How can you use your knowledge of leadership models and styles to interact with emerging leaders?
- How can you use your knowledge of the models and styles to help emerging leaders analyze situations in the workplace and develop strategies to address them?

Developing the Knowledge and Skills to Mentor Emerging Leaders

Clinical training continues beyond formal education. Typically, experienced leaders have seen more cases with a variety of disorders and extent of deficits than emerging clinicians. Acquiring

Table 10–1. Summary of Leadership Theories and Models

Theory/ Model	Key Style Factor
Trait	Leaders are naturally endowed with superior characteristics and traits.
Behavior	Leaders are characterized by how they behave regarding employee orientation, production, and relations.
Contingency/ Situational	Leaders apply different styles in different situations.
Transformational	Leaders use the strength of their vision to change expectations, perceptions, and motivations to achieve common goals. This leader is typically thought of as a *charismatic* leader.
Servant	Leaders seek to serve and improve the lives of their employees, customers, and stakeholders. Servant leadership is thought to be an extension of transformational leadership and requires decision makers to lead from a moral perspective that guides their behavior.
Authentic	Leaders exhibit a positive moral perspective characterized by high ethical standards that guides their decision making, behaviors, values, beliefs, and actions.
Ethical	Leaders demonstrate ethical conduct through their personal actions and promote such conduct in their subordinates.

Source: Adapted from Walston, S. L. (2017). *Organizational behavior and theory in healthcare.* Chicago, IL: Health Administration Press.

additional knowledge and skills should be an ongoing process for both experienced and emerging leaders. The knowledge and skills necessary for clinical training and supervision are transferable skills that can be used to mentor emerging leaders. The America Speech-Language-Hearing Association's Board of Directors and its Ad Hoc Committee on Supervision listed the knowledge, skills, and abilities required of individuals who supervise clinical training (ASHA, 2013):

- Knowledge of clinical education and the supervisory process, including teaching techniques, adult learning styles, and collaborative models of supervision;
- Skill in relationship development, including the creation of an environment that fosters learning;
- Ability to communicate, including the ability to define expectations and engage in difficult conversations;
- Ability to collaboratively establish and implement goals, give objective feedback, and adjust clinical education styles when necessary;
- Ability to analyze and evaluate emerging leader's performance, including gathering data, identifying areas for improvement, assisting with self-reflections, and determining if goals are being achieved;
- Skill in modeling and nurturing clinical decision-making, including (a) using information to support clinical decisions and solve problems and (b) responding appropriately to ethical dilemmas;
- Skill in fostering professional growth and development;
- Skill in making performance decisions, including the ability to create and implement plans for improvement and to assess the emerging leader's response to these plans; and
- Ability to adhere to the principles of evidence-based practice and to convey research information to clinicians.

The Council on Academic Programs in Communication Sciences and Disorders developed supervisory courses that address these supervisory competencies (Council on Academic Programs in Communication Sciences and Disorders [CAPSCD], 2017). Virtual clinical supervision courses are also offered by ASHA and at national and state association conventions. The supervisory courses are a systematic approach to training and preparing clinical educators. Clinical educators often become mentors for graduate students during clinical practica and beyond. Clinical educators also establish and maintain a rapport with emerging leaders years after graduate school and may help shape their clinical decision-making and life skills. Therefore, the supervisory skills that experienced clinicians acquire are some of the same skills needed for effective mentoring. transfer to the skills necessary to become an effective mentor.

In addition, experienced leaders should self-assess their cultural competency and ability to interact with individuals with diverse backgrounds. ASHA has numerous resources to expand multicultural competency that experienced leaders can access to self-reflect and discover any biases they may have regarding the culture of their mentees. Philippe (2011) states that:

> Mentoring is relationship oriented and intends to create a safe environment. In order for participants to openly share professional and personal issues, there must be safety. A safe place exists only where there is trust. It takes a mental shift to believe that this particular person who differs in many ways will not judge . . . or try to hurt the emerging leader. (paragraph 4)

Establishing a cross-cultural relationship and rapport takes time, as well as positive experiences between the experienced and emerging leaders.

Establish Rapport that Fosters Cross Cultural and Generational Communication with Emerging Leaders

As the face of America changes, the number of culturally and linguistically diverse (CLD) health care professionals must increase to address to needs of a diverse society (Bush & Windmill, 2008; Bush, Scott, Lemmon & Cluster, 2014). A recent census profile indicated that by the year 2050, the minority population in the United States will expand by at least 44% (U.S. Census Bureau, 2008), which signifies an increase in the number of individuals from culturally and linguistically diverse backgrounds. This will require audiologists, speech-language pathologists, and other allied health professionals to augment their cultural competency. Suarez-Balcazar and Rodakowski (2007) concluded that "becoming culturally competent is an ongoing contextual, developmental, and experiential process of personal growth that results in professional understanding and improved ability to adequately serve individuals who look, think, and behave differently from us" (p. 15). Similarly, establishing relationships with emerging leaders from culturally diverse backgrounds also require cultural considerations. Mentors should consider implicit biases and any personal stereotypes when mentoring individuals of another culture. Implicit bias is not intentional or conscious in nature (Wyatt, Laderman, Botwinick, Mate, & Whittington, 2016). It extends beyond racism to social factors such as age, gender, sexual orientation, gender identity, disability status, and physical appearance attributes like height and weight. Though it may be automatically activated and unintentional, self-awareness helps overcome individuals' implicit biases. The majority of research on implicit bias relates to the relationship between health care practitioners and patients; however, these same strategies apply to interacting with emerging leaders who are from culturally and linguistically diverse backgrounds and to all who are marginalized by society. Harvard University's Project Implicit offers a test to assess implicit or unconscious bias (https://implicit. harvard.edu/implicit/takeatest.html). Below are strategies that experienced leaders can use to reduce implicit bias ("How to Reduce," 2017):

- Stereotype replacement: Recognizing that a response is based on stereotype and consciously adjusting the response
- Counter-stereotypic imaging: Imagining the individual as the opposite of the stereotype
- Individuation: Seeing the person as an individual rather than a stereotype (e.g., learning about their personal history and the context of their leadership abilities)
- Perspective taking: Putting yourself in the other person's shoes (e.g. imagine being the only or one of a few African American or Latina at management level meetings or in an SLP/ Audiology Department in the workplace)
- Increasing opportunities for contact with individuals from different groups: Expanding one's network of friends and colleagues or attending events where people of other races, ethnicities, gender identities, sexual orientation,

and other groups may be present. Begin by asking two questions, "What breaks your heart?" and "What makes you come alive?"

- Partnership building: Reframing interactions as one between collaborating equals, rather than between a high-status person and a low-status person.

Instructing emerging leaders requires that experienced leaders establish a strong rapport and trust with them. This is especially true for cross cultural mentoring (Phillipe, 2011). Establishing and maintaining rapport with emerging leaders in a variety of contexts is of utmost importance for effective communication and mutual understanding. Emerging leaders' initial experience with establishing professional rapport occurs during the collegiate experience with professors, instructors, and clinical supervisors. Though professors and clinical supervisors mentor students to acquire educational and clinical competence, all students will not receive structured leadership development. Professors may collaborate and establish rapport with small groups of students on structured collaborative research or professional projects, involving activities that receive a grade. These early interactions set the parameters for later interactions with mentors (cross-cultural or intergenerational) in the workplace. Likewise, a positive or negative relationship with individuals of a different cultural background may color emerging leaders' future interactions with individuals from that cultural background. As a result, it may take individuals longer to feel comfortable using an open dialogue with an authentic voice that represents their true thoughts and feelings (Hutchins, 2018). Establishing rapport includes setting guidelines for professional interactions, types of interactions, and modes and frequency of communication. This is particularly important in cross generational interactions between experienced and emerging leaders, where experienced and emerging leaders may have different ways of communicating (e.g., virtually versus in person), modes of communication (e.g. text versus calls), or different ideals of professional interactions (e.g., in a coffee house versus an office). Miscommunication may occur as a result of these different ways of conveying messages from the sender to the receiver. Thus, mentors and mentees should discuss the basics of communication, and delineate mutual guidelines. For example, an experienced leader may prefer not to take phone calls or receive text messages after a certain hour of the day. If these basics of communication are negotiated at the beginning of the relationship, there will be no confusion about the guidelines for exchanging communication. Furthermore, experienced leaders should be flexible and open to using new or unfamiliar modes of communication. Perhaps consider meeting at a coffee house instead of the office a few times, or using FaceTime or Skype as opposed to a phone call a time or two. One simple compromise can result in building trust from the onset of the relationship.

Professional interactions can occur during research meetings, presentations, and professional project or tasks. The modes of communication can include phone calls, emails, texts, and video conferencing (Facetime, Skype, Zoom). Experienced and emerging leaders should discuss and agree on the mode of communication that best suits both individuals. There should also be a discussion regarding the frequency of communication. Specifically, decide if communication should occur on a weekly, monthly or quarterly basis. Provide guidelines for the latest time in the evening that each may contact the other by phone or text. The types of interactions will vary based on the nature of the leadership training. Meetings can occur in the office, a library, or coffee shop based on the nature of the relationship. Discussing these guidelines openly and at the beginning of interactions help develop emerging professionals' soft skills for current and future communication and interactions. It also sets parameters for future interactions with their mentors while emphasizing soft skills (e.g., accountability, refraining from calling or texting after a specific time).

Guidelines for Meetings with Emerging Leaders

Emerging leaders should be encouraged to initiate meetings at the frequency they and their mentors agreed upon. It is challenging for experienced leaders to continuously bear the responsibility for setting up meetings. After all, they are typically busy individuals who volunteer their time and expertise to assist mentees with professional development. Initiating meetings empowers emerging leaders to take ownership of their leadership development and alleviates experienced leaders of the burden so they can attend to countless other professional and personal obligations. It creates an environment that respects both in-dividuals' time and professional obligations and shows that emerging leaders are engaged as well as committed to their development process. Time is the one commodity in life that cannot be replaced; therefore, it is absolutely priceless. Emerging leaders initiating meetings avoids wasting irreplaceable time and energy on individuals who do not truly want to advance in their leadership development. Experienced leaders should save their energy and time for individuals who are truly dedicated and focused on self-improvement and cultivating leadership acumen. Though experienced leaders may recognize potential in an individual's ability, emerging leaders must also recognize their own potential and actively engage to acquire additional leadership skills.

Structured Interaction with Emerging Leaders

Developing a productive relationship requires that both individuals spend quality time during structured interactions. Structured interactions include collaborating on various tasks, projects, or committee assignments, which provide opportunities to achieve a common goal. During these interactions experienced leaders needs to be flexible and receptive to completing the task in a way that differs from their own style. Mentees may use technology in an innovative way or have a different opinion from their mentors and remaining receptive to using their suggestions will validate their ideas. Experienced leaders should also make a concerted effort to talk to mentees about current events and activities to develop their soft skills (e.g., small talk). Provide positive reinforcement for tasks throughout collaborations and for completed projects that are delivered on time and that meet or exceed expectations. Many millennials work for the satisfaction of contributing toward the greater good of an organization and positive reinforcement is the stimulus that fuels their actions (Myers & Sadaghiani, 2010).

Miscommunication Between Experienced and Emerging Leaders

Miscommunication during intergenerational interactions can leave emerging leaders with the feeling that the experienced leader is critical, unsupportive, and unreceptive to their ideas. McCready (2011) cited examples of intergenerational differences (e.g., technology usage, communication styles, and perceived work ethics) that can occur in the workplace. Explicitly discussing these differences is necessary to ensure a positive, productive, and supportive environment for emerging leaders while avoids frustrating experienced leaders during the mentoring process. While there are many differences between generations, there also many similarities.

In general, emerging leaders strive to cultivate positive relationships. Most individuals want positive interactions (especially interactions with leaders) that support the mission of the organization as well as their personal missions (Building Movement Project, 2010). Creating a positive environment for leadership growth helps experienced leaders and emerging leaders establish a relationship built on trust and respect. Sharing a personal mission to improve leadership ability (at any stage) sets the tone for a healthy environment in which both individuals can cultivate their leadership abilities. The sharing of information will inform the experienced leader of the emerging leader's mission and their envisioned future. Experienced leaders benefit from positive interactions with emerging leaders, which will break negative stereotypes that have been fostered in the media and print about millennials, fostering a view of them as individuals with a wide range of attributes suited for today's global society (Myers & Sadaghiani, 2010). The experienced leader's sharing affords the emerging leader the opportunity to glean knowledge (be it institutional knowledge or personal reflection) that is not accessible in journal articles or elsewhere online.

Informal Interactions with Emerging Leaders

Informal encounters, such as one-on-one interactions in a coffee house, restaurant, or between sessions at professional meetings, help develop emerging leaders' soft skills. It is during these interactions that emerging leaders solidify their ability to process, synthesize, and apply new information gleaned from collaborative projects; effectively communicate professionally related content; and make small talk with other professionals in their experienced leader's professional circle. Indeed, informal interactions truly help establish solid networking skills that continue to grow throughout a experienced leader's career. Therefore, informal interactions become the basis of building emerging leader's professional career; specifically, it offers access to collaborative opportunities and experiences unavailable within the four walls of their workplace, that can catapult their careers further and faster.

Providing Feedback to Emerging Leaders

During interactions with emerging leaders, explicitly explain the rationale and benefits of feedback (positive and corrective action). In addition to providing suggestions for improvement, emerging leaders may want to know the experienced leader's reasons why suggestions for improvement are made. In fact, it is quite natural to want to know the rationale behind the experienced leader's decisions and learn from the extensive or historical knowledge used to find creative solutions. Experienced leaders should not be offended; instead, take pride that the emerging leaders want to know why decisions are made because it shows that the mentee is not willing to be blindly led by others. Experienced leaders who do not provide a rationale for suggested changes may encounter emerging leaders who voice their opinions why the feedback is not accurate or even why organizational policies should change or evolve. This represents a generational difference between Millennials and Baby Boomers because Millennials expect open communication during feedback and may voice dissenting opinions which may be perceived as disrespectful (McCready, 2011; Myers & Sadaghiani, 2010).

Millennials have openly voiced their opinions from a very young age during interactions with parents, adults, and online platforms (McCready, 2011; Myers & Sadaghiani, 2010). Furthermore, young women are encouraged to voice their opinions and question status quo. Speech-language pathology is a female dominated profession. As such there may be differences in communication styles between women of differing generations. It is not bad to voice dissenting opinions; however, it is advantageous to guide the emerging leader on ways to use their voice within an organizational culture. The *Voice Positioning System: 7 Ways to Harness Your Power and Master Your Influence* by Dr. Katrina Hutchins (2018), is based on a phenomenon referred to as organizational silence. In her description of organizational silence Hutchins says, "the choice not to speak up, but rather withhold opinions and ideas about issues or concerns at work, is within itself the most simplistic description of organizational silence" (p. 18). This research on organizational silence revealed that before beginning a career, women expressed feelings of powerlessness, apprehension, and submission when silenced. Women may be silenced by society norms or standards. After becoming employed, the women felt resigned, resentful, and a need for self-preservation. In contrast, when their authentic voices were embraced within the workplace, the women had feelings of self-regulation, self-determination, and self-inclusion. This research showed that silencing a person's voice leads to many negative emotions that trap and prevent the sharing of ideas and opinions. Similarly, the "Me Too" movement emphasizes the life-changing realization that women's (and men's) voices matter and will be heard, thereby breaking previous societal silence surrounding sexual abuse (Ohlheiser, 2017). Likewise, the mission of the Black Lives Matter network is to build local power and intervene in violence inflicted on Black communities. It has given a voice to African Americans who have been silenced by being systematically killed, oppressed, or marginalized for expressing their opinions and using the power of their voice (Black Lives Matter, n.d.). Imagine if leaders spoke quickly, definitively, and powerfully to denounce slavery, sex trade, or the Holocaust. Millennials, who are the next generation of emerging leaders, are characterized as socially conscious individuals who use their voices to authentically express their opinions and stand in their truth (Building Movement Project, 2010). Therefore, questions from emerging leaders should not be viewed as disrespectful, but as a sign that they want to know the thought process for deriving an answer or position on a topic. This is a definitive sign that they are using critical and analytical thinking skills to "voice their opinions, harness their power and master their influence" (Hutchins, 2018, p. 52).

Constructive Criticism and Emerging Leaders

Providing constructive criticism is a natural, though sometimes uncomfortable, part of leadership development training. Experienced leaders should preface constructive criticism with positive comments, which set the tone for emerging leaders to accept and reflect on the constructive criticism for future improvement. This may include providing genuine positive feedback on their propensity to develop into an impressive leader. Follow up with specific constructive criticism and convey the information in a nonjudgmental manner. Provide specific examples related to tasks, not the person. Encourage emerging leaders to reflect on feedback and develop strategies to overcome their weaknesses. Then, work with them to devise an action plan for improvement.

When emerging leaders implements the plan, provide positive feedback regarding the improvement in performance (if it indeed improves). List the importance and functionality that the newly gained strength (i.e., former weakness) brings to the workplace or team. Mentees should intellectually know and emotionally feel that you are invested in their professional growth, as opposed to continuously pointing out weaknesses. Providing positive feedback after implementing an action plan leaves mentees with a sense of pride in achieving a goal with their mentor's support. This fosters a positive relationship that affirms that their mentor is truly invested in an emerging leader's future growth and upwards mobility!

Periodic Pulse Checks

After emerging leaders implement action plans for improving weaknesses, conduct periodic *pulse checks*. Pulse checks are impromptu interactions with emerging leaders via phone calls, emails, or text messages. This intermittent communication should comprise open-ended questions (e.g., "How are you?" or "How are your plans progressing?"). It lets emerging leaders know that you are there for support, assistance, and guidance, and that you are invested in their continued success. Over time, continuous interactions with them will enable you to gauge the level of support that an individual needs to be successful. As a result of these interactions, emerging leaders should feel comfortable initiating conference calls, lunch, or formal meetings to update you on their progress or obtain additional suggestions or assistance. Pulse checks help to move relationships past constructive criticism and into the realm of positive affirmation of success.

Developing Hard Skills

To fully develop emerging leaders' abilities, experienced leaders should set expectations for hard skills. Hard skills are teachable skills or abilities that are easy to quantify (Doyle, 2018). Hard skills are straightforward and outlined in the Council of Academic Accreditation in Audiology and Speech-Language Pathology Standards (2017) for students who matriculate through academic programs. They are documented for each student during graduate matriculation for both disciplines. These are the core academic skills that an individual learns in order to obtain the Certificate of Clinical Competence (CCC) awarded by the ASHA. Specific examples of hard skills include the following:

- Establish a clear set of program goals and objectives that student must meet to acquire the knowledge and skills needed for entry into independent professional practice.
- Establish a clear process to evaluate student achievement of the program's established objectives.

- Offer opportunities for each student to acquire the knowledge and skills needed for entry into independent professional practice, consistent with the scope of practice for audiology or speech-language pathology, and across the range of practice settings.

Acquisition of hard skills ensure that student leaders and emerging professional leaders truly know their craft. Thus, student leaders must study to truly learn information, as opposed to studying to pass course exams in graduate school or an entry level professional exam (e.g., Praxis II; National Examination in Speech-Language Pathology or Audiology). Ultimately, emerging leaders must be able to proficiently apply information learned in the academic setting in clinical practice. Later in life, emerging leaders have opportunities to lead groups of professionals. Leaders with subpar clinical skills have difficultly leading. Lack of clinical skills in leadership can engender a lack of respect from staff because the leader is perceived as inept. Once respect is lost, it is very difficult to regain.

Developing Soft Skills

Soft skills are personal attributes and abilities that allow individuals to work well with others. Soft skills are necessary for success in clinical practice, the workplace, and in life. Some important soft skills that leaders in CSD must acquire are listed below:

- Positive attitude
- Effective communication skills
- Problem-solving and critical thinking skills
- Collaborative skills
- Accepting constructive feedback
- Civility
- Dependability
- Compassion

Assisting emerging leaders with developing soft skills is often an issue of debate or contention because some individuals feel that soft skills are inherent as opposed to teachable. It is worth developing soft skills in emerging leaders to improve interaction and communication with clients and coworkers, and there are multiple ways to do so. One of the most effective strategies is to emphasize common interest with emerging leaders. For instance, having one shared ultimate goal in mind to develop the necessary skills to become successful. Instead of initially bringing up areas of weakness in terms of soft skills, the conversation should revolve around attributes required to become an effective leader. Emerging leaders are smart, savvy, and able to apply the information to their own life. If not, explicitly state areas they need to strengthen when the opportunity arises. An opportunity will arise because the area of weakness will become an issue in the workplace or during the emerging leader's tenure with an organization. Emphasize that developing the absent or weak soft skill can help emerging leaders rise to greater heights of success. The ultimate shared goal is for emerging leaders to achieve success through the assistance and mentorship of the experienced leader.

Developing Emotional Intelligence

Daniel Goleman conducted ground-breaking research on emotional intelligence; in his book *Emotional Intelligence* (1995), Goleman described numerous examples of people with a high intelligence quotient (IQ) who floundered in leadership positions, while individuals with modest IQs exhibited leadership acumen. Essentially, the qualities commonly associated with leadership, such as intelligence, decisiveness, determination, and vision, are necessary for success; however, these characteristics are not sufficient to successfully lead an organization at a transformational or servant leadership level. Highly effective leaders must also have a solid degree of emotional intelligence. Goleman (1995) showed an explicit link between a leader's emotional intelligence and measurable business results. As such, emerging leaders must develop emotional intelligence to successfully interact in the workplace.

Emotional intelligence is the ability to identify your emotions, understand what the emotions are telling you, and know how they affect the people around you" (Goleman, 1995, 2004). It also requires accurate perception of others' emotions. Emotional intelligence enables relationships to operate effectively by gauging and respecting each other's emotions. Goleman (1995; 2004) states that the primary characteristics of emotional intelligence are motivation and social skills like self-awareness, self-regulation and empathy, which also happen to be characteristics of successful leaders. Emerging leaders must learn to regulate their emotions and apply problem-solving strategies to resolve issues and manage others' emotions in order to cheer up or calm down other individuals (Goleman, 1995, 2004).

High emotional intelligence enables leaders to motivate others to complete tasks on time and remain focused on outcomes, rather than capitulate when criticized by others. Table 10–2 provides definitions and examples of characteristics individuals with high emotional intelligence possess.

Training and professional coaching may ameliorate emotional intelligence of the emerging leader. Experienced leaders who find their mentees lacking in emotional intelligence, can provide resources for the mentee to self-assess, such as online quizzes to identify areas of weakness. Some online quizzes even provide recommendations on how to manage emotions and readings to improve emotional intelligence through practice and feedback. Mentors who establish a strong rapport with emerging leaders, can provide feedback and emerging leaders should be receptive to the feedback. Below are some online resources (e.g., websites, quizzes, and videos) for emerging leaders to assess and develop their emotional intelligence.

Assessments of Emotional Intelligence:

- https://www.mindtools.com/pages/article/ei-quiz.htm
- https://globalleadershipfoundation.com/geit/eitest.html
- https://www.ihhp.com/free-eq-quiz/

Development of Emotional Intelligence:

- https://www.ted.com/talks/daniel_goleman_on_compassion/transcript?language=en
- https://www.youtube.com/watch?v=pt74vK9pgIA

Table 10-2. Characteristics of Individuals with High Emotional Intelligence (EI)

EI Component	Definition	Examples*
Self-Awareness	Knowing one's emotions, strengths, weaknesses, values, and goals—and their impact on others	A clinician knows tight deadlines bring out the worst in him. So, he plans his time to get work done well in advance.
Self-Regulation	Controlling or redirecting disruptive emotions and impulses	When a team botches a presentation, its leader resists the urge to scream. Instead, she considers the possible reasons for the failures, explains the consequences to the team, and explores solutions with them.
Motivation	Being driven to achieve for the sake of achievement	A manager at a rehab company sees productivity declining for three consecutive quarters. Doctors are not referring new patients. She decides to learn from the experience—and engineers a turnaround.
Empathy	Considering others' feelings, especially when making decisions	A child who is Hispanic is diagnosed with a genetic disorder. The mother, who speaks limited English, attends a meeting alone with the treatment team. The interpreter shares that the mother is distraught about the new diagnosis. The team leader stops the meeting and informs the mother that the meeting will reconvene when her husband or other family member is present for emotional support.

continues

Table 10–2. *continued*

El Component	Definition	Examples*
Other Social Skills	Managing relationships to move people in a desired direction	A clinical director wants to move to an electronic record keeping system to improve billing efficiency and meet new federal guidelines. The clinical director seeks buy-in from clinicians in the practice and the company's owner. The new electronic record keeping system is adopted.

*Examples adapted to reflect to communication sciences and disorders.

Sources: Adapted from Goleman, D. (1995). *Emotional intelligence.* New York, NY: Bantum Books.

Goleman, D. (2004, January). What makes a leader? *Harvard Business Review* [E-book]. Retrieved from https://scopetraining.com.au/wp-content/uploads/2015/10/Daniel-Goleman-What-makes-a-leader-article-R0401H-PDF-ENG.pdf

- https://scopetraining.com.au/wp-content/uploads/2015/10/Daniel-Goleman-What-makes-a-leader-article-R0401H-PDF-ENG.pdf
- https://liveboldandbloom.com/02/self-awareness-2/emotional-intelligence-workplace

Developing Networking Skills

Developing networking skills help emerging leaders progress further and faster in their careers. Valuable information is gleaned from relationships with professionals who have different experiences than one's own. Networking extends beyond having the gift for gab in social situations. It means cultivating ongoing, mutually beneficial relationships with individuals who work together to achieve professional goals. Forbes Media (2013) recommends the following basic networking skills to immediately improve the emerging leaders' skills:

- Get off the computer (or cell phone or iPad). Many relationships begin on social media or professional sites liked LinkedIn or ASHA Community. However, it is vital to connect in person to establish an authentic professional relationship (Forbes Media, 2013). Connect with individuals by asking them to lunch, or coffee, or attending a speech-language pathology or audiology event together.
- Forget you're working. Emerging leaders should engage and give their complete attention after being introduced. They should immerse themselves in the conversation and get to know individuals, as opposed to thinking about possible work-related benefits of knowing an individual. Thinking about how an individual can benefit their career may distract them from interacting in an authentic manner.
- Set goals. Set goals related to networking such as, "I will get three business cards at the state association convention," or "I will set up two coffee dates with new contacts at the next ASHA convention." These types of goals nudge emerging leaders to get offline and connect in person.
- Mind your manners. Tried and true societal manners matter. Encourage emerging leaders to (1) listen more than talk, (2) be thoughtful during interactions, and (3) be generous with their time whenever possible. New relationships can flourish with great manners and sink with rudeness.
- Elevator pitch skills matter. Emerging leaders should be able to succinctly sell their career interests, such as what they are doing career wise. For instance, they may be interested in working with specific types of clients (e.g., preschoolers who are medically fragile, individuals who have experienced a neurological infarct resulting in a stroke, children receiving school-based services).
- Play to your weaknesses. Determine networking skills weaknesses. These weaknesses will vary for each individual. If an emerging leader does not follow up with

new contacts, encourage setting a phone reminder to contact individuals within a week of meeting them.
- Don't hang on to business cards. After meeting an individual during a networking event, immediately enter the information from business cards into a cell phone or email contacts. This eliminates the possibility of losing a business card with phone numbers and contact information.

Establishing and maintaining authentic relationships with renowned individuals help emerging leaders meet their professional goals. In all professional relationships, mutual passion for a specific discipline coupled with an experienced leader's desire to positively influence the emerging leaders' career sets the emerging leader on an upward trajectory.

Establishing Professional Goals

Obtaining any level of success requires the ability to have a vision, set obtainable goals, achieve the goals, and recalibrate to set additional goals. This process should include evaluating the extent to which the goals are met. Therefore, goals should be specific, measurable, attainable, and time bound in order to ensure that the mentees meet the goals. Encourage emerging leaders to explore a variety of paths to achieve their goals and provide feedback. This creates a clear vision or road map for an emerging leader and encourages them to take ownership of their goals. Emerging leaders should develop an action plan with timelines to reach their goals. Emerging leaders might set a goal but fail to explore ways to reach the goal. For example, if the goal is to become a rehabilitation director within five years, an emerging leader may not consider all of the steps they must take to achieve this goal. For instance, an experienced leader may suggest breaking down the goal of becoming a rehabilitation director into specific subgoals. If mentees are unsure of the steps required to reach the goal, the experienced leader can introduce them to a rehabilitation director to seek insight, research the qualifications of rehabilitation directors, and use all of the information obtained to develop subgoals. Alternatively, encourage them to think critically about the goal and ways to achieve it; then discuss the strengths of the plan and revise the steps as needed to achieve the desired outcome. Discuss the emerging leader's progress toward goals with them and ways that you can assist them in reaching their goals. Experienced leaders may need to point out that some goals take months to complete, whereas other goals may take years; explain that therefore, they must exercise tenacity and perseverance to reach some goals. Discussions also serve to hold individuals accountable for acquiring the skills they need and actively working toward achieving their professional goals. In fact, accountability for achieving skills can be included in professional goals that emerging leaders set, which will serve to guide them toward their life vision. It takes tenacity and perseverance to achieve their vision!

Empowering Emerging Leaders to Accomplish Goals

Empower emerging leaders to accomplish their goals by discussing how far they have gotten toward achieving the goals. Offer support and encouragement during formal meetings and informally in emails, texts, or even on social media (blogs, Facebook, or Twitter accounts if you feel comfortable) or professional media accounts (e.g., LinkedIn or ASHA Connect). Provide opportunities for emerging leaders to connect with other professionals who can assist with reaching their goals. Explicitly state that the contact information (e.g., phone number, email) is for their use only. Emphasize that it is not professional to share the contact information with others without consent. Provide collaborative opportunities to research, present, write documents (reports, articles, book chapters, position statements) or serve as an assistant during a professional leadership opportunity. During such an experience, emerging leaders can observe experienced leaders' processes, strategies, procedures, and leadership abilities over time. This may be an extensive time commitment, so provide this opportunity only for individuals who are dependable, have exceptional abilities, and most importantly, are committed to their own personal and professional growth. As an experienced leader, you should be able to ascertain which individuals are amenable to feedback and have the perseverance to continue the project through completion. Prior to beginning a project, explicitly state the nature of the opportunity, guidelines, and timelines to set expectations and ensure that you complete the project with the professional relationship intact.

Resources for Developing Leadership

ASHA has an array of leadership development and mentoring programs to cultivate the next generation of leaders. These programs are designed to allow leaders to give back to the profession through volunteering and to develop speech-language-pathologists' and audiologists' leadership skills. Most recently, ASHA began a Leadership Academy (American Speech-Language-Hearing Association, n.d.) that prepares individuals to deepen their knowledge based on their interest and time availability via assessments, webinars, mentoring, blogs, and podcasts. The Council on Academic Accreditation in Communication Sciences and Disorders (CAPCSD) also has a Leadership Academy that builds the leadership abilities of individuals who work in higher education. The following resources can be found on ASHA's website and within the ASHA Community referred to as the "Leadership Academy" (Table 10–3).

ASHA is taking great care to develop the next generation of leaders by supporting these programs as pipelines to leadership. It is especially timely that ASHA is considering ways to diversify leadership through initiatives within its Office of Multicultural Affairs. A diverse workforce or volunteer group includes individuals of different races, sexual orientations, as well as other differentiating factors, and brings a unique thought process and outlook to organizations that can improves their economic performance, increase productivity, improve creativity (Walston, 2017).

Paying It Forward

It is imperative that emerging leaders internalize the concept of paying it forward to continue the cycle of propagating the seeds of leadership that will ultimately catapult organizations or

Table 10–3. Resources for Leadership Development

Leadership Development and Mentoring Programs	Brief Description	Website
ASHA's Leadership Development Program	A year-long program for ASHA members with leadership potential. This program has focused subsections for different professions (SLPs, audiologists, health care professions).	https://www.asha.org/About/governance/Leadership-Development-Program/
Council on Academic Programs in Communication Sciences & Disorders (CAPCSD) Leadership Academy	An academy for individuals considering academic (e.g., college and university) leadership positions or who are newly engaged in academic leadership to develop their knowledge and skills in the area of leadership.	http://www.capcsd.org/?s=Leadership+Academy&search=Search
ASHA's Leadership Mentoring Program (pilot program)	Part of ASHA's continued efforts to develop ASHA's volunteer leadership and a diverse pipeline of future leaders for the profession.	https://community.asha.org/Go.aspx?MicrositeGroupTypeRouteDesignKey=fdb2f4a1-4a4d-4c6d-bcde-f767260ab6fb&NavigationKey=2d13686b-cd17-421b-88e2-ae5ed31692cb
ASHA's Student to Empowered Professional (S.T.E.P) Mentoring Program	An online mentoring program where mentees and mentors communicate to address a short- or long-term goal via email, phone, text, or Facebook.	https://www.asha.org/Students/mentoring/step/AboutSTEP/

continues

Table 10–3. *continued*

Leadership Development and Mentoring Programs	Brief Description	Website
ASHA's Minority Student Leadership Program (MSLP)	A leadership development program established for undergraduate seniors, master's students, and Doctor of Audiology (AuD) students enrolled in communication sciences and disorders (CSD) programs, and PhD students pursuing a research doctoral degree.	https://www.asha.org/Students/MSLP-Award/
ASHA's Students Preparing for Academic-Research Careers (SPARC) Award	An award that aims to cultivate student interest in pursuing a PhD and a career as a faculty-researcher in CSD.	https://www.asha.org/students/SPARC-Award/
ASHA's Mentoring Academic-Research Careers (MARC)	Supports PhD students, postdoctoral fellows, and junior faculty in obtaining and succeeding in faculty–researcher positions in CSD.	https://www.asha.org/students/gathering place/marc/

Data Sources: American Speech-Language-Hearing Association Community (2018), Leadership Academy; Council on Academic Programs in Communication Sciences and Disorders (2018), Leadership Academy.

professions to another level. Include opportunities for emerging leaders to participate in peer mentoring for others to create an efficient pipeline of emerging leaders. For instance, organizations can offer leadership development programs to create pathways to leadership and opportunities for emerging leaders to assist the next group of individuals who want to strengthen their leadership skills. Emerging leaders should be expected to help others. Encourage them to develop an altruistic spirit if they do not have one innately. Outgrow your job! As a consummate professional and experienced leader, you have done a great job developing emerging leaders' skills and abilities. Gradually decrease your assistance and encourage them to become independent. Do the job of developing emerging leaders so well that they do not need you as frequently over time. Give them the tools they need to lead and achieve the next level of their career. Bask in the manifestation of your efforts. Encourage them to continue honing their networking skills. Encourage them to check in with you as needed and to share the joys of attaining a goal or garnering an award. An exceptional emerging leader will surpass your accomplishments because you have done an amazing job of developing their leadership skills. Be secure in the knowledge that their accomplishments are a byproduct of your exceptional leadership development skills. Quickly squelch any feelings of jealousy or resentment. After all, emerging leaders achieved their level of success at a quicker pace as a result of your mentorship, commitment (time and resources), professional networks or connections to other leaders, and assistance with obtaining their goals. John Maxwell, a preeminent author and lecturer on leadership development, considers experienced leaders who led extremely well for a long period of time as creators of leadership legacies within the organization as the pinnacle of leadership (Maxwell, 2011). Maxwell (2011) asserts that, high level leadership improves an organization and produces a positive environment for everyone. During their prime, experienced leaders should impact and develop as many emerging leaders as possible for future succession planning within the organization and industry; as a result, this contributes to the future viability and sustainability (Maxwell, 2011). Experienced leaders who choose to help develop emerging leaders will touch, change, and positively impact countless lives while creating a legacy of leadership!

References

American Speech-Language-Hearing Association (2013). *Knowledge, skills and training for consideration for individuals serving as supervisors* [Final report, Ad Hoc Committee on Supervision]. Retrieved from http://www.asha.org

American Speech-Language-Hearing Association (n.d.). *Leadership academy*. Retrieved from https://community.asha.org/leadership academy/home

Building Movement Project. (2010). *What works? Developing successful multigenerational leadership*. Retrieved from http://www.building-movement.org/pdf/what_works.pdf

Bush, D., Scott, D., Lemmon, R., & Cluster, N. (2014, November). *Speech-language pathology and physician assistant students' perceptions of cultural competency*. Poster session presented at the American Speech-Language Hearing Association Convention, Orlando, FL.

Bush, D., & Windmill, E. (2008). Diversity in the audiology profession. *Audiology Today, 20*(6), 40–51.

Black Lives Matter (n.d.). About. Retrieved from https://blacklivesmatter.com/about/

Council on Academic Accreditation in Audiology and Speech-Language Pathology (2017). *Standards for accreditation of graduate education programs in audiology and speech language pathology*. Retrieved from https://www.asha.org/uploadedFiles/ASHA/Article/Accreditation-Standards-Graduate-Programs.pdf

Doyle, C. (2018). *Hard skills vs. soft skills: What's the difference?* Retrieved from https://www.thebalancecareers.com/hard-skills-vs-soft-skills-2063780

Forbes Media (2013). Improve your networking skills—Right now. *Forbes.com*. Retrieved from https://www.forbes.com/sites/thesba/2013/01/24/improve-your-networking-skills-right-now/#3195ef3a6e3e

Goleman, D. (1995). *Emotional intelligence*. New York, NY: Bantum Books.

Goleman, D. (2004). What makes a leader? *Harvard Business Review*. Retrieved from https://scopetraining.com.au/wp-content/uploads/2015/10/Daniel-Goleman-What-makes-a-leader-article-R0401H-PDF-ENG.pdf

Hutchins, K. (2018). *The voice positioning system: 7 ways to harness your power and master your influence*. Columbia, SC: Re-Source Solutions.

Maxwell, J. (2011). *The 5 levels of leadership: Proven steps to maximize your potential*. New York, NY: Hatchette Book Group.

McCready, V. (2011). Generational issues in supervision and administration. *The ASHA Leader, 16,* 12–15.

Myers, K. K., & Sadaghiani, K. (2010). Millennials in the workplace: A communication perspective on millennials' organizational relationships and performance. *Journal of Business and Psychology, 25*(2), 225–238.

Ohlheiser, A. (2017, October 19). The woman behind 'Me Too' knew the power of the phrase when she created it—10 years ago. *Washington Post.* Retrieved from https://www.washingtonpost.com/news/the-intersect/wp/2017/10/19/the-woman-behind-me-too-knew-the-power-of-the-phrase-when-she-created-it-10-years-ago/?noredirect=on&utm_term=.16bcb8dff97c

Philippe, M. Y. (2011, May 19). Cross cultural mentoring: A case for inclusiveness in action. *Profiles in Diversity Journal.* Retrieved from http://www.diversityjournal.com/4454-cross-cultural-mentoring-a-case-for-inclusiveness-in-action/

Suarez-Balcazar, Y., & Rodakowski, J. (2007). Becoming a culturally competent occupational therapy practitioner: Practical ways to increase cultural competence. *OT Practice, 12*(17), 14–17.

U.S. Census Bureau. (2008). *Press release CB08-123.* Available from www.census.gov/Press-Release/www/releases/archives/population/012496.html.

Walston, S. L. (2017). *Organizational behavior and theory in healthcare.* Chicago, IL: Health Administration Press.

Wyatt, R., Laderman, M., Botwinick, L., Mate, K., & Whittington, J. *Achieving health equity: A guide for health care organizations* [Institute for Healthcare Improvement white paper]. Cambridge, MA: Institute for Healthcare Improvement.

End Notes

The journey of writing and collaborating on this book has been a learning process and I hope reading it is an instructive journey for others. The information regarding professional preparedness in a career leading to management and leadership is invaluable to me as I work with and train others. The notion of where there are gaps and how to fill them and the personal maturity and supports needed to develop leadership are two of the most valuable lessons in my opinion. The vast amount of insight and resources required to analyze oneself in a growth industry such as communications cannot be overestimated.

Availability of more continuing education and business practice courses in graduate curricula may help prepare young clinicians on the move. In the growing industry of rehabilitation, it is imperative that young leaders know how to invest in a facility's mission and vision and how to establish metrics for a department's growth and longevity. Being able to present trends and comparisons in a concise forward-thinking manner is just one of the skills that business leaders need, but may not have studied intensively.

Many of the leadership attainment strategies are shared decision-making in corporations with multi-layered administrations where hands-on learning may not be possible. However, insightful managers know what information senior management is looking for and will have the facts and figures required for internal department strategizing. The fast-paced environment of medical economy legislation, the growing demographic of high-need populations, and the increased demographic of populations with diverse needs are just a few of the challenges facing even small to midsize operations.

To survive and function, departments must show consistent positive productivity measures and have systems in place to prevent shortfalls. The ability to perceive and predict threats to an organization's livelihood is an invaluable asset to managers in growth departments, such as speech rehabilitation and education. The more effective a leader is, the better chance for survival and growth in an increasingly competitive marketplace, and for functional and appropriate outcomes for consumers of services.

Effective and efficient operations are the cornerstone of principled management. Management sets a very high personal and professional bar for young, and even more seasoned professionals, especially in a field that is relatively new and has been historically female-dominated. Traditional speech communications specialists may have been in the workplace for fewer years than specialists tend to be now. With this change we should expect to see more and more female executives taking their place in the boardroom and in the highest levels of administration. Developing one's self and one's skill set, and taking advantage of workplace or online learning opportunities, for example, will be critical to get and keep positions of leadership in the industry. Individuals may require time to be spent on learning and growth, with extra commitment to specialized academies and workshop opportunities after the work week is over.

A new area of demand for competitive managers in senior organizations is more detailed performance metrics and preparation to visualize future goals, trends, and resources. One of the most useful tools for seeking and retaining the top-level positions in tomorrow's organizations is specialized books that offer insight from established leaders in various communication industries and settings.

Index

Note: Page numbers in **bold** reference non-text material.

235

Z

Zeitgeist, defined, 150
Ziskin, Ian, 153

Zone of proximal development (ZPD), 123
ZPD (Zone of proximal development), 123–124